DBT® TEAMS

GUILFORD DBT® PRACTICE SERIES
Alan E. Fruzzetti, *Series Editor*

This series presents accessible, step-by-step guides to essential components of dialectical behavior therapy (DBT) practice. Delving deeply into different aspects of DBT implementation—phone coaching, validation, chain analysis, family interventions, and more—series volumes distill the latest clinical innovations and provide practical help based on sound DBT principles and good science.

Phone Coaching in Dialectical Behavior Therapy
Alexander L. Chapman

Chain Analysis in Dialectical Behavior Therapy
Shireen L. Rizvi

DBT® Teams: Development and Practice
Jennifer H. R. Sayrs and Marsha M. Linehan

DBT® Teams

Development and Practice

Jennifer H. R. Sayrs
Marsha M. Linehan

Series Editor's Note by Alan E. Fruzzetti

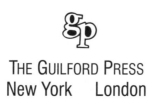

THE GUILFORD PRESS
New York   London

Library of Congress Cataloging-in-Publication Data

Names: Sayrs, Jennifer H. R., author. | Linehan, Marsha M., author.
Title: DBT^q teams : development and practice / Jennifer H.R. Sayrs, Marsha M.
   Linehan.
Other titles: Dialectical behavior therapy teams
Description: New York : The Guilford Press, [2019] | Series: Guilford DBT^q
   practice series | Includes bibliographical references and index.
Identifiers: LCCN 2019015458| ISBN 9781462539819 (paperback) | ISBN
   9781462539826 (hardcover)
Subjects: LCSH: Dialectical behavior therapy. | BISAC: MEDICAL / Psychiatry /
   General. | SOCIAL SCIENCE / Social Work. | PSYCHOLOGY / Emotions.
Classification: LCC RC489.B4 S24 2019 | DDC 616.89/142—dc23
LC record available at https://lccn.loc.gov/2019015458

About the Authors

Jennifer H. R. Sayrs, PhD, ABPP, has served as a research therapist on three of Marsha Linehan's dialectical behavior therapy (DBT) clinical trials and as a DBT adherence coder on several trials. As a trainer for Behavioral Tech, she provides a wide range of DBT workshops in the United States and around the world. She is Director of the DBT Center at the Evidence Based Treatment Centers of Seattle (EBTCS), where she provides DBT to adults, adolescents, and families. The DBT Center was one of the first DBT teams in the nation to be awarded Program Certification by the DBT-Linehan Board of Certification. Dr. Sayrs is also a founding member and Executive Director of EBTCS. She is a board member of the American Board of Cognitive and Behavioral Psychology, a specialty board of the American Board of Professional Psychology.

Marsha M. Linehan, PhD, ABPP, the developer of DBT, is Professor of Psychology and of Psychiatry and Behavioral Sciences and Director of the Behavioral Research and Therapy Clinics at the University of Washington. Her primary research interest is in the development and evaluation of evidence-based treatments for populations with high suicide risk and multiple, severe mental disorders. Dr. Linehan's contributions to suicide research and clinical psychology research have been recognized with numerous awards, including the 2017 University of Louisville Grawemeyer Award for Psychology and the 2016 Career/Lifetime Achievement Award from the Association for Behavioral and Cognitive Therapies. She is also a recipient of the Gold Medal Award for Life Achievement in the Application of Psychology from the American Psychological Foundation and the James McKeen Cattell Award from the Association for Psychological Science. In her honor, the American Association of Suicidology created the Marsha Linehan Award for Outstanding Research in the Treatment of Suicidal Behavior. She is a Zen master and teaches mindfulness and contemplative practices via workshops and retreats for health care providers.

Series Editor's Note

Dialectical Behavior Therapy—Then and Now

This outstanding book on DBT team consultation is the third book in the Guilford DBT® Practice Series, which was developed to meet the increasing needs of practitioners to learn how to practice dialectical behavior therapy (DBT) well—in an adherent and competent way. DBT was developed originally for suicidal and/or self-harming patients with borderline personality and related disorders. While the DBT treatment manual (Linehan, 1993a), the revised *DBT Skills Training Manual* (Linehan, 2015b), and the *DBT Skills Training Handouts and Worksheets* (Linehan 2015a) provide therapists with the entire treatment protocol, other aspects of the treatment—chain analysis, validation, phone coaching, family interventions, consultation team, and effective use of dialectical strategies, to name a few—have developed considerably beyond the original treatment manual. It is for this reason that we developed this series, with the support of Dr. Marsha M. Linehan, to help practitioners enhance and refine their skills and deliver DBT to their patients more effectively, according to present DBT standards and practices.

When the young psychologist Marsha Linehan and her colleagues at the University of Washington developed DBT in the 1980s, it was not at all clear if the treatment would be successful, in terms of both treatment efficacy for people who are chronically suicidal and self-harming (typically referred to as having borderline personality disorder, or BPD), for whom the treatment was developed, and acceptance and adoption for use by the therapeutic community, who long had struggled to treat people with these problems. In order to understand how the accessible guides in this series enhance the literature and promote adherence to current DBT principles and practices, we must first show how they fit into the overall structure of DBT treatment and the treatment context for BPD and related problems that has evolved over time.

Looking back 30 years or more, it is stunning to see the impact Dr. Linehan's work has had on the field. Before her work became widely disseminated and accepted, suicidal and/or self-harming people with BPD faced rampant stigmatization, a sense of hopelessness about recovery, and a complete absence of empirically supported treatments. Needless to say, people with DBT faced a bleak prognosis. At the time, DBT was available only in a small clinic at the University of Washington. There was no treatment manual or skills manual; there were no clear ways to teach, disseminate, or implement the treatment effectively.

Where are we now? Stigma has been significantly reduced, hope has increased, there is a general recognition among professionals that BPD and related problems are treatable (although there is still a long way to go), and an impressive volume of studies demonstrate strong support for DBT's efficacy and effectiveness. There is a widely read treatment manual (Linehan, 1993a), and both an original (1993b) and enhanced and updated skills manual (2015a, 2015b). Well-trained teams in outpatient, residential, hospital, and other settings treat thousands of people every day with DBT, not only across the United States but in dozens of countries and on every continent. Many of these treatment providers have demonstrated both their commitment and their abilities by becoming certified as DBT therapists, which requires rigorous demonstration of their skills as DBT providers. In addition, other effective treatments, generally also nonpejorative toward people with BPD and related difficulties, have been empirically established or are under development.

Moreover, applications and adaptations of DBT have been successfully developed for a host of problems other than BPD per se (i.e., other severe problems related to emotion dysregulation) and across a variety of treatment—and, more recently, prevention—settings. It's not a surprise that Dr. Linehan was recently featured as one of the 100 "Great Scientists" of all time ("Great Scientists," 2018).

DBT is an *integrative* treatment that includes a whole set of interventions (modes and functions of treatment). DBT includes not only individual therapy but also multiple other modalities that serve different functions in treatment, such as group skills training, telephone coaching, family interventions, and an ongoing consultation team. DBT integrates the techniques and scope of acceptance-oriented therapies (e.g., support, warmth, encouragement) with the strategies and precision of behavior therapies and emotion science (e.g., precise treatment targets, scientific analysis of behavior [emotions, thoughts, actions]) and focuses on psychological and social skills as *solutions* to a range of problems. Dozens of controlled studies support the effectiveness of DBT in creating safety, stability, and self-control while minimizing treatment dropout, as well as improving mood, self-esteem, relationships, family, school and job functioning, and so forth. Largely due to stable outcomes and reduced relapse, costs of DBT compared to alternative treatments are also significantly reduced in the long term.

The DBT Model

The treatment model views *emotion dysregulation* as the core of a variety of emotional, cognitive (thinking), relational, identity (self-concept), and behavioral problems. Emotion dysregulation increases or exacerbates behavioral dysregulation (out-of-control actions, including impulsivity), cognitive dysregulation (trouble thinking and problem solving), interpersonal dysregulation (difficulties in relationships), and self-dysregulation (problems with self-esteem, identity, negative self-views). Consequently, many common co-occurring problems (suicidal and nonsuicidal self-injury, depression, anxiety, eating disorders, posttraumatic stress disorder, substance abuse, aggression, problems in relationships, etc.) are similarly understood either as dysfunctional attempts to regulate emotion or as natural consequences of chronic emotion dysregulation. The overarching goal of DBT is to help people create lives worth living by helping them learn psychological and social skills to regulate, or manage, their emotions—earlier in treatment tolerating and re-regulating secondary emotions, and later in treatment identifying, accurately labeling, allowing, expressing accurately, and managing primary emotions. Much of the treatment is built around these principles.

Chronic and severe emotion dysregulation is hypothesized to result from an ongoing *transaction* between the person's emotion vulnerabilities and ongoing invalidation from others in the social and family environment, which often promotes self-invalidation as well. Emotion vulnerability is influenced by temperament, conditioning, and present biological disposition resulting from learning and current circumstances and manifests as emotional sensitivity and reactivity, along with often slow return to emotion equilibrium. Invalidating responses can take a variety of forms, from the obviously critical and emotionally abusive to well-meaning misunderstandings that occur because of temperamental differences, inaccurate expression, or miscommunication between people and their family members and others.

Five Core Functions of Comprehensive DBT

DBT consists of components or modes that address the five essential functions of treatment:

1. Help people learn new psychological, emotional, and social/relationship skills, typically via skills training groups (skill acquisition).

2. Help people generalize those skills to their real, everyday lives, in situations that have elicited less skillful responses in the past, which includes detailed planning, *in vivo* coaching, and practicing skills in the "real" world (skill generalization).

3. Help people collaborate on their treatment targets and enhance their motivation to replace overlearned dysfunctional behaviors with more skillful alternatives, primarily through individual psychotherapy, and also in other ways, depending on treatment setting (motivation to replace dysfunctional behaviors with skillful alternatives).

4. Help people manage their social and family relationships to build better relationships and elicit more support, understanding, and validation and help family members become more validating and supportive in return (structure the social and family environments to promote improvements).

5. Provide ongoing support, validation, problem solving, and skill building for therapists to enhance their motivation and skills through regular team consultation meetings (increase skills and motivation for DBT providers). This is the topic of the present book.

DBT Skills

Learning key psychological, emotional, and social skills is believed to be central in helping patients learn to regulate their emotions, build satisfying relationships, and thrive. These include skills to:

1. Increase attention control and nonjudgmental awareness and build a more positive self-concept or identity (mindfulness).

2. Understand emotions, increase positive emotions, decrease vulnerability to negative reactions, accept negative emotional experiences, and change negative emotional experiences (emotion regulation skills).

3. Build empathy and improve relationships while balancing assertion with self-respect (interpersonal skills).

4. Tolerate highly distressing experiences without doing things impulsively that increase dysregulation overall (distress tolerance skills).

5. Balance competing goals, interests, and perspectives and build cognitive and emotional flexibility (dialectics, or the middle path, along with "wise mind").

Over time, some additional skills have become part of the DBT lexicon, such as dialectical and validation skills for patients and their families, specific skills for people with substance use problems, and so on (cf. Fruzzetti, Payne, & Hoffman, in press; Miller, Rathus, & Linehan, 2007; Rathus & Miller, 2015).

Of course, principles of learning are at the core of any behavior therapy, including DBT. In particular, there are three overlapping phases of learning: (1) the acquisition phase, in which the basics of the skill are learned, typically in skills training groups designed to be optimal learning environments; (2) the strengthening phase, in which the person practices the skill, typically in planned ways, in groups or with the therapist or at home; and (3) the generalization phase, in which the person's skill has become robust enough that the person can employ it when needed in their life, often spontaneously. Of course, in addition to the teaching/training and coaching that occur in skills training groups and in individual sessions, in outpatient settings *in vivo* coaching can help to generalize skills (mostly by text or telephone) and manage between-session problems.

Acceptance and Validation

Throughout DBT, treatment providers strive to understand and validate the primary emotional experience of their patients, along with other valid behaviors, and help clients validate themselves. We do not validate things that are not, in fact, valid. This is a complex task, learning to discriminate the valid aspects of any given behavior from the invalid ones. For example, certain impulsive and/or destructive behaviors (e.g., self-harm, substance use) are typically primary targets for change because they are invalid ways to solve problems or enhance quality of life in the long term. Yet, they are valid in the sense that they do often "work" to reduce, avoid, or escape painful negative emotional arousal, albeit briefly. Understanding and validating what is valid, even in the most dysfunctional behavior, is a key therapeutic activity that helps the client feel understood (validated), increases motivation for change, builds the therapeutic relationship, and thus increases collaboration for change. Consequently, therapist validation not only has value in itself (feeling understood, cared about, etc.), it also helps regulate the person and promotes change.

Change, Problem Solving, and Behavior Therapy

Within a therapeutic context based on understanding, acceptance, and validation, the therapist targets dysfunctional behaviors for change, pushing patients to substitute skillful alternatives for the problematic reactions and dysfunctional behaviors for which they sought treatment. Utilizing a carefully constructed treatment target hierarchy, DBT therapists and the DBT team can employ all the components of learning and behavior therapy: (1) careful assessment, using chain analysis; (2) development of solutions on the chain and replacement of dysfunctional "links" in the chain that led to a dysfunctional or undesired behavior with a skillful alternative (this includes learning skills, noted above); (3) behavioral rehearsal and other commitment strategies to foster the difficult change process; and (4) all the techniques of behavior therapy to help the person actually use the skill when needed (e.g., stimulus control, reinforcement/contingency management, exposure and response prevention).

Dialectics

Balancing acceptance and validation with change, problem solving, and behavior therapy is complicated, and there are no algorithms to guide us because each context is unique. Rather, the therapist must balance these dialectically in the service of effectiveness. Every strategy in DBT has an "opposite" of equal value that must be considered and balanced in order to help people change in the ways they want to change. Just as acceptance and validation must be balanced with change and problem solving, intervening on behalf of clients is balanced by consulting with clients to empower them to intervene on their own behalf; communicating in a warm, genuine, and caring way must be balanced with irreverence, insistence, and matter-of-fact communication; and emotion must be balanced with reason (and vice versa).

Interventions in the Social and Family Environments

Although an important component of DBT from the beginning, social and family interventions are areas that have shown enormous growth and development since the first wave of DBT was developed and implemented. For example, fully developed applications of DBT have been shown to be effective with parents, couples, and families, and in school systems, and are being used to prevent the development of emotion dysregulation problems or to intervene early to help clients avoid full-blown problems related to emotion dysregulation. All of these efforts utilize the core principles of DBT, but of course have expanded the strategies and techniques to be effective in these new domains. Their growth and development are a positive testament to the coherence and effectiveness of DBT from the beginning.

What DBT Is and What It Is Not

Given the strong empirical foundation for DBT, it is no surprise that many clinicians want to offer DBT as part of their therapeutic toolbox. However, DBT is complex and requires considerable time, effort, and dedication to learn well. So, it is also not surprising that a wide range of treatments are offered under the DBT "label," but are of varying DBT quality. This is confusing for consumers at best, and of course fraudulent at worst. Imagine if a surgeon thought, "I've never had the training to do this procedure, but I read a little bit about it, so I can advertise myself as an expert in it." No one would want this surgeon performing a procedure on them. Fortunately, a certification process for DBT therapists, and their DBT teams, is now underway. This is a significant positive development both for people who need treatment (they will know what they are getting) and for DBT therapists (they will have objective measures that show they are doing excellent work).

How This Book Series Fits into the Development of DBT

DBT is, at least metaphorically, a living, breathing, and always growing and evolving treatment. It expands and changes in a dialectical manner. We use the therapy according to the model (the "thesis" or "proposition"); when something is not working well, DBT therapists innovate within the treatment ("antithesis" in which we employ theory and science to develop something new). In response to data and research findings about these innovations, we find some things work and others do not; ultimately, some new strategies or interventions become established and integrated with the old (synthesis, now established treatment), and stay that way until a situation arises in which they do not work well, and then further innovation (further antitheses) is engaged.

The original text (Linehan, 1993a) remains relevant and wise and includes an enormous amount of thoughtful and effective guidance. DBT has evolved since 1993 to include many more things (applications in new settings, extensions of principles and strategies, new skills, etc.) that could not have been anticipated at the time the book was written. This book series presents DBT as it is today, synthesizing the old and the new, built on the original treatment manual.

For example, the first book in this series (Chapman, 2019) focuses on telephone consultation with clients. This idea of coaching suicidal and self-harming clients by telephone between sessions was an innovative notion and was greeted by many therapists as a potential barrier to learning and practicing DBT. Were clients going to abuse their phone privileges, intrude on therapists' lives, and make never-ending demands on therapists' time? Chapman shows how to observe therapeutic limits, coach but not provide treatment, and use phone time to effectively advance treatment. He also presents detail about how coaching might differ for teens compared with adults, and other aspects of phone coaching that have emerged over time with a great deal of innovation and empirical evaluation.

Similarly, Shireen Rizvi's book on chain analysis (2019) provides details and nuance well beyond early iterations of DBT. Chain and solution analyses are the core method of understanding clients' experiences and problems and thus provide opportunities for validation. In addition, they are the foundation for change strategies, allowing the therapist and client to "swap out" dysfunctional thoughts and reactions and "swap in" skills as alternatives. Doing one or more chain and solution analysis is part of every individual DBT session. Rizvi expertly highlights not only the ins and outs of doing chains and solutions but also the complex dialectical process that goes into completing a successful chain and solution analysis, including validating key behaviors on the chain, shaping, managing treatment-interfering behavior, and developing and implementing solutions that are effective and efficient.

This current book fills in many gaps in the important area of how to build and run an effective DBT team. Most treatment teams in mental health services serve as vehicles for information exchange and/or administrative activities. The DBT team eschews this approach entirely in favor of a team in which genuineness is a key ingredient and in which there are clear targets for the team: (1) enhancing therapist motivation via support, validation, etc., and (2) improving therapist skills via problem solving, teaching/learning, practice, or rehearsal (e.g., role plays). Both of these targets are in the service of providing adherent DBT.

Formulating clear goals and targets, a flexible but useful structure, and a clear process for a consultation or treatment team are among the innovative contributions that Marsha Linehan made as she developed DBT. Indeed, the structures and processes that Jennifer Sayrs and Marsha Linehan lay out for us in this book not only are incredibly helpful for DBT therapists and teams, but easily could be employed with few or no adaptations to many other treatments. The authors highlight that the DBT team is a community of therapists and provide guidance on how to build a warm, genuine, and effective community that meets the needs of its members for support and growth. Rather than give rigid rules, teams use ordinary DBT principles to develop flexible, often sophisticated structures and processes to guide practitioners, providing teams with many choices to fit their particular clinical situations.

One reason for a well-functioning treatment team in DBT is that many clients, especially at the beginning of treatment, have severe problems and improvement can take months. Thus, the potential for therapist burnout is high. Moreover, in difficult clinical situations the therapist's emotions can run high. Sayrs and Linehan guide us through multiple solutions to prevent the burnout that can result from these highly stressful situations. High emotion can interfere with cognitive processing, memory, and problem solving, which means that therapists can become "de-skilled" at times. Meeting colleagues on a DBT team helps therapists manage these difficult clinical situations as they emerge, preventing burnout and likely improving treatment outcomes. Sayrs and Linehan provide multiple guidelines and examples for how to do this effectively.

The authors, ultimately, have put together a truly expert guide that provides everything we need to start, build, and manage an effective consultation team. They present clear principles and offer practical examples to show how to frame problems and how to generate solutions.

They also continue the tradition in this series of providing sophisticated yet practical help in how to use updated practices in DBT while also honoring the standards and traditions of DBT (e.g., Linehan, 1993a) and, at the same time, exploring more fully what it means to create and maintain an effective DBT team. For example, Linehan (1993a) identified six original team agreements. In this book, Sayrs and Linehan go on to identify a dozen more team agreements that are likely to help organize the team in a variety of ways.

Jennifer Sayrs is an expert in DBT, having completed her doctoral work at the University of Nevada, Reno, where she practiced DBT for her entire tenure there and then in a postdoctoral fellowship at the University of Washington, where she worked directly with Marsha Linehan. Jennifer is a founding member and Executive Director of the Evidence Based Treatment Centers of Seattle and spent 7 years as Director of Training before assuming her current role as Director. She has a reliable DBT adherence rating and has taught DBT extensively in the United States and internationally.

Marsha Linehan has had a profound impact on the field of psychotherapy in general, as her work developing DBT has had significant influence on how we think about and treat borderline personality disorder, emotion in cognitive-behavioral therapy (CBT), emotion dysregulation, treatment teams, and countless other problems and phenomena.

This book is essential reading for both novice DBT therapists and well-established clinicians. It employs the principles of DBT throughout

while providing sound guidelines and practical examples and suggestions, and incorporates new learning, research, and new standards for
DBT teams that have become established over the past 25 years. Moreover, this book could be invaluable to therapists who practice CBT or
other modalities who are interested in addressing provider burnout and/
or want treatment teams to accomplish more than simply exchange
information. And, of course, the material in this book is entirely consistent with core DBT competencies, adherence in DBT (necessary for
certification as a DBT therapist), and Linehan's initial treatment manual
(1993a). The entire series intends to augment, rather than replace, earlier core DBT manuals (Linehan, 1993a, 2015a, 2015b), and this book
truly enhances and extends our thinking about and practices on DBT
teams. Each book in this series, including this one, illustrates many new
developments guided by both clinical innovation and sound research
that constitute DBT today.

ALAN E. FRUZZETTI, PhD

References

Chapman, A. L. (2019). *Phone coaching in dialectical behavior therapy*. New York:
Guilford Press.

Fruzzetti, A. E., Payne, L., & Hoffman, P. D. (in press). Dialectical behavior therapy
with families. In L. A. Dimeff, K. Koerner, & S. L. Rizvi (Eds.), *Dialectical
behavior therapy in clinical practice: Applications across disorders and settings* (2nd
ed.). New York: Guilford Press.

Great scientists: The geniuses and visionaries who transformed our world. (2018).
Time (Special Edition). New York: Time, Inc.

Linehan, M. M. (1993a). *Cognitive-behavioral treatment of borderline personality disorder*. New York: Guilford Press.

Linehan, M. M. (1993b). *Skills training manual for treating borderline personality disorder*. New York: Guilford Press.

Linehan, M. M. (2015a). *DBT skills training handouts and worksheets* (2nd ed.). New
York: Guilford Press.

Linehan, M. M. (2015b). *DBT skills training manual* (2nd ed.). New York: Guilford
Press.

Miller, A. L., & Rathus, J. H., & Linehan, M. M. (2007). *Dialectical behavior therapy
with suicidal adolescents*. New York: Guilford Press.

Rathus, J. H., & Miller, A. L. (2015). *DBT skills manual for adolescents*. New York:
Guilford Press.

Rizvi, S. L. (2019). *Chain analysis in dialectical behavior therapy*. New York: Guilford
Press.

Acknowledgments

Jennifer H. R. Sayrs: First and foremost, I want to thank my two DBT mentors, Marsha Linehan and Alan Fruzzetti. I joined my first DBT team with Alan in 1994 and remained on that team for several years. I then joined Marsha's training team as a postdoctoral fellow and later her research teams. The experience of working closely with both of these mentors, including supervision, modeling, and mentorship, has been profound. It is difficult to put into words the impact they both have had on me. I learned DBT and so much more: mindfulness, precision, compassion, dedication, and perseverance are just a few examples. From both of them, I gained an ability to help a significant number of people who deeply needed help. And writing this book with Marsha has been a very meaningful experience; I am grateful for her wisdom, guidance, and encouragement. I am so happy to have both Marsha and Alan as mentors, colleagues, and friends.

I feel profound gratitude for Sarah Reynolds, Jennifer Waltz, and Sona Dimidjian, who read an earlier version of this book and provided thoughtful, important feedback. Their efforts improved this book immensely. Lizz Dexter-Mazza and Shireen Rizvi were also tremendous sources of support and guidance. These amazing women are dear friends who were invaluable in getting me through this process.

Thank you to my DBT team at Evidence Based Treatment Centers of Seattle (EBTCS). Whenever I feel stuck in a session, I think, "Thank goodness for my team!" They embody the dialectic of acceptance and change, providing intense support while making each other better providers at every meeting. Having such tremendously dedicated, skilled, compassionate colleagues has made it possible for me to continue providing DBT for as long as I have. My most recent DBT colleagues include Joanna Berg, Karen Berlin, Kjersti Braunstein, Jessica Chiu, Ashley Connors, Peter Doyle, Sarah Huffman, Alex Ivey, Briana McElfish, Kaimy Oehlberg, Alisa Pisciotta, Rachel Partin, Natalie Stroupe, and Joanna Watson; a special thank you to Blair Kleiber, who has gone the extra mile to help me run our team. There have also been many prior team members who remain important to me. I want to thank Beatriz Aramburu, who was my teammate for 18 years. Our DBT team is truly a lifeline for me each and every day.

I am also grateful to my other colleagues at EBTCS. I am particularly thankful for David Lischner, who has supported our DBT program since its inception and has been especially supportive of me through some challenging times. Travis Osborne, Elizabeth Lagbas, and all of my amazing colleagues at EBTCS are inspiring! Every day I am impressed by their dedication and skill. I love working with all of them.

My skilled and compassionate colleagues at Behavioral Tech have taught me so much. They have provided a professional home to me for many years, and I am grateful to know all of them. I'd like to give a special thank you to Tony DuBose and André Ivanoff, who have provided me so many opportunities to do such meaningful work. Thank you to the Society for Dialectical Behaviour Therapy, and particularly Michaela Swales and Christine Dunkley, for their support as well.

To my own individual clients, I am honored that they allowed me to work so closely with them. Their vulnerability, strength, and determination are inspiring. Seeing the changes that were made possible by DBT and our work together has been a profound experience for me. There truly was a transaction: they have impacted me as much as our work impacted them. They have shaped me into being a better therapist and bring a very important sense of meaning, care, and joy to my life. I have grown tremendously from our work together.

I am inspired and moved by the hard work of the many providers and teams I have worked with as a colleague, supervisor, and trainer. So much of what is in this book comes from their successes, challenges, and reflections. I have learned so much from my experiences with them, for which I am grateful.

I would like to thank Kitty Moore at The Guilford Press for seeing the value in this project and for her guidance and patience throughout. Thank you to other members of the Guilford team as well, including Anna Nelson, Carolyn Graham, Robert Sebastiano, Philip Holthaus, Judith Grauman, and Carly DaSilva.

Thank you to Erica; without her guidance and care, this book would not have been completed.

Most importantly, thank you to my family. This project took several years from start to finish. My husband, daughters, and parents provided emotional and practical support, fun, and a lot of patience, and I am grateful to all of them.

Marsha M. Linehan: I would like to thank Jennifer Sayrs, who had the fabulous idea of our writing this book together. Working with Jennifer has been so meaningful to me, especially as I see her determination and patience to make this book the best it can be.

I have led several DBT consultation teams during my long career—the ones for clinical trials usually ran for 5 years; the one in which I train graduate students and postdoctoral fellows has lasted over 15 years. I am grateful to the many students and postdoc trainees who have made our DBT team an invaluable learning community and effective at improving the delivery of care to our clients. I am also grateful to our clinical supervisors who gave countless hours to supervising our trainees and who made our DBT training program such an outstanding one. I want to especially thank the following supervisors: Beatriz Aramburu, Adam Carmel, Jessica Chiu, Emily Cooney, Caroline Cozza, Angela Davis, Lizz Dexter-Mazza, Michelle Diskin, Clara Doctolero, Dan Finnegan, Andrew Fleming, Vibh Forsythe-Cox, Bob Goettle, Melanie Harned, Michael Hollander, Kelly Koerner, Janice Kuo, Liz LoTempio, Shari Manning, Annie McCall, Jared Michonski, Erin Miga, Andrea Neal, Kathryn Patrick, Adam Payne, Ronda Reitz, Sarah Reynolds, Magda Rodriguez, Jennifer Sayrs, Sara Schmidt, Trevor Schraufnagel, Stefanie Sugar, Jennifer Tininenko, and Randy Wolbert.

I thank Katie Korslund and Ron Smith for their wise counsel and Corey Fagan for teaching the requisite clinical skills to students before they joined our DBT training program. I am grateful to the Behavioral Research and Therapy Clinics staff whose ongoing support has enabled me to direct our center, conduct research, do clinical work, teach students, and disseminate DBT.

Contents

Purchasers can download and print enlarged versions
of the handouts at *www.guilford.com/sayrs-forms*
for personal use or use with their DBT team (see
copyright page for details).

DBT Teams

An Introduction

Dialectical behavior therapy (DBT®) is a principle-driven, modular, cognitive-behavioral treatment originally developed for chronically suicidal individuals diagnosed with borderline personality disorder (BPD). Most typically consisting of a combination of individual psychotherapy, group skills training, telephone coaching, and a therapist consultation team, DBT has been shown through randomized controlled trials (RCTs) to be efficacious for BPD, with emerging evidence suggesting that it is useful with a wide range of other problems related to emotion dysregulation (see Rizvi, Steffel, & Carson-Wong, 2013, for a review of this research).

This book assumes at least a basic knowledge of DBT. There are many books and resources on DBT; some follow DBT principles and theory closely, and some do not. To learn about DBT, we recommend starting with the DBT treatment manuals (Linehan, 1993, 2015a, 2015b), which are the manuals used in the RCTs on DBT. They will provide the best basis for learning DBT, and for understanding this book. We refer to these treatment manuals throughout this book.

The Functions of DBT

As a comprehensive treatment, DBT has several functions or jobs it must serve in order to be effective with the high-risk, challenging clients, with multiple, chronic problems, it was designed to treat. As described in the original treatment manual (Linehan, 1993), they include:

- Increasing capability (i.e., teaching skills; typically accomplished via skills training group).

- Increasing motivation (i.e., arranging variables such that the client is more likely to engage in effective behavior and less likely to engage in ineffective behavior; most often addressed in individual therapy).

- Generalizing skills to the client's environment (i.e., utilizing strategies to get the new behavior to occur in the client's own environment; this usually includes phone calls and texts with the provider outside of session as well as homework assignments, and can include additional strategies such as listening to recordings of the previous session at home).

- Structuring the environment (i.e., there are a variety of ways to arrange the environment such that it supports DBT; this may be done with the individual therapist, a family therapist, a case manager, and/or other providers or strategies).

- Building team members' motivation, capability, and adherence to the treatment manual (i.e., "hold the therapist inside the treatment"; Linehan, 1993, p. 101; providers typically address this function within a DBT team).

In RCTs focused on the efficacy of DBT, all of these functions were addressed in some way (most often in the standard arrangement described above; however, there is flexibility in how these functions are met). In order to be considered "full" or "comprehensive" DBT, each of these functions must be addressed.

The DBT Team

The concept of a "treatment team" in DBT started in research trials, where a team approach was utilized to ensure that therapists followed the treatment manual and other research protocols. While this started as a practical strategy, it quickly became clear that the team was an *active* component of the treatment. It was evident in the early development of DBT that, in dealing with very-high-risk, emotionally dysregulated clients, providers could become so frightened of suicide risk that they were prone to make decisions based on emotion, rather than on the treatment plan. DBT providers also at times became frustrated or burned out with clients who engaged in aversive interpersonal behavior. Providers' own personal problems (e.g., health issues, relationship problems) at times also impacted the treatment they provided. Clients also inadvertently reinforced nontherapeutic interventions and avoidance, and even punished effective strategies. Overall, providers inadvertently drifted from the treatment manual, without realizing they had drifted. It became abundantly clear that having team members who provided each other with support, encouragement, and validation while doing this difficult work, along with feedback and guidance regarding adherence to the manual, was essential in keeping these providers on track. It was due to this discovery that DBT formally included the treatment team as an essential component.

Despite its importance, DBT teams have received relatively less focus in books, workshops, and webinars compared to training on DBT individual therapy and skills. This dearth is notable, as the team is considered the fulcrum of the treatment, a place where team members can recalibrate and center themselves to provide the best treatment possible. After training and consulting to many DBT programs around the world, we determined that while DBT programs were highly motivated to have a team, they were left with many questions and challenges. Teams can be incredibly helpful, supportive, and comforting; they can also cause frustration and stress when problems are not managed effectively. In other words, teams take work to establish and maintain. The importance of teams, coupled with the lack of instruction and information, led us to identify the need for a manual for the DBT team.

This book is designed to provide guidance for developing and maintaining a DBT team. It is written for any DBT provider (or non-DBT provider) who wishes to create a DBT team, or who already has a team and would like to further enhance its functioning. When we refer to "team members," this is not limited to individual therapists or skills trainers, but is meant to address anyone who is a member (or wishes to become a member) of a DBT team and is providing an intervention with DBT clients. At times we refer to team members as "therapists" (as in "a community of therapists"), providers, or clinicians; these terms are meant to include *any* member of a DBT team. Team membership is discussed further in Chapter 8.

The Functions of the DBT Team

The overarching goal of the DBT team is to help team members provide the best DBT possible. As far as we know, adhering to the DBT manual is the most effective way to deliver DBT. Adherence to the DBT manual has been a required component of many of the RCTs on DBT (see Rizvi et al., 2013, for examples of such RCTs), and fidelity has been shown in other treatments to be associated with improved client outcomes (e.g., DeRubeis & Feeley, 1990), as well as greater staff retention when fidelity monitoring is presented as supportive consultation (Aarons, Sommerfeld, Hecht, Silovsky, & Chaffin, 2009). To meet this goal of adherence, Linehan (1993) described the DBT team as having two functions, as mentioned above: to enhance both the motivation and the capability of DBT providers.

1. *Motivation.* Teams work to maximize providers' motivation to deliver effective treatment to their clients. "Motivation" can refer to several things: First, teams can enhance providers' willingness to provide DBT. Teams provide a "safe haven," a confidential environment where team members are comfortable being vulnerable, and where they share and receive support. Teams help each member feel cared about, an "insider" in a group of like-minded individuals. Teams can also help each member balance clients' needs with their own limits, to help prevent burnout. Teams can even be fun! Just as in DBT treatment, motivation also means lining up the controlling variables such that effective provider behaviors are reinforced, and ineffective behaviors are minimized. The DBT team can enhance motivation by helping to set up the environment such that each team member is steered toward the most effective action possible. This includes noticing when members engage in problematic avoidance and making sure they are reinforced for approaching a difficult intervention; it may also mean helping a teammate regulate any intense emotion that interferes with treatment delivery.

2. *Capability.* Teams also aim to increase each member's capability. This refers to the skill with which the overarching treatment is delivered, as well as each DBT strategy and protocol. This goal also includes ongoing monitoring to be sure team members are providing DBT, helping team members learn how to improve their interventions, and highlighting when a member may have drifted from the treatment manual.

The team might recommend seeking consultation, finding a training or treatment manual, or any number of strategies to make the treatment as precise and effective as possible.

This manual will focus on how to attain both of these functions, such that DBT team members are motivated and capable of providing the most effective DBT possible.

Not a Traditional Team

The idea of providers meeting in a team is nothing new. Teams have a long history in mental health, in settings such as hospitals, residential treatment centers, and other places where providers meet daily or weekly to discuss client care. These teams allow for individuals from various disciplines to work together, share information, inform each other of progress and problems, coordinate care, and provide a unified treatment to clients. These teams traditionally focus primarily on the client, not the provider. Additionally, these teams are typically not considered formal parts of the treatment; rather, they are practical, administrative solutions to make sure providers are consistent and informed.

Coordinating care is, of course, extremely important. However, there are several ways in which DBT teams are quite different from traditional consultation teams (Sayrs, 2019). First, a core concept of the DBT team is that of community. A DBT team is considered a *community of therapists treating a community of clients.* In other words, DBT team members work together, as a team, to treat *all* of their clients. This creates a different sense of team, "we are all in this together," as well as a different level of investment in each other's clients: each team member is invested in helping each teammate provide excellent care to all the clients associated with the team, and in this way, every teammate is treating every client. This means that if a provider is struggling to provide effective care due to burnout, frustration, or life events, the team moves in and helps in some manner, because their teammate and the team's client is struggling. If a teammate notices that a member has drifted from the manual or is being shaped into ineffective behavior with a client, it is essential to highlight this problem, because every member of the team is "treating" this client. This idea of community is taken so seriously that if one DBT provider has a client die by suicide, all members of the team say they had a client die by suicide. It is not "their" client; it is "our" client.

DBT is also set apart from traditional teams in that the DBT team focuses on *therapy for the therapist,* rather than directly on clients. Clients are, of course, discussed in team, but the primary focus is how to help *team members* adhere to the manual, improve their motivation and skills, and enhance the effectiveness of their treatment. In other words, the team provides DBT strategies aimed at the *provider,* to address any obstacles that might arise in client care. For example, in a traditional team, a provider might say, "My client called me too much this weekend," and the team would focus on the client's behavior. In a DBT team, the provider would change the focus: "I started to feel frustrated at all the calls I got from one client this weekend. I could use some help getting my frustration level down, and deciding what to do about the calls." The team then focuses on providing suggestions and recommendations, along with support and validation, to help the provider manage the situation as effectively as possible.

In order to provide effective therapy for the therapist, a DBT team also requires a different level of vulnerability than traditional teams. The team emphasizes, in a confidential environment, being open about mistakes and uncertainty, in order to obtain support and help. To get this type of help, DBT team members openly discuss challenging or unsuccessful moments in therapy, even when they involve shame, frustration, or other difficult emotions. It may also involve sharing personal events that could affect therapy (while still observing their own limits).

And finally, DBT teams are different from traditional consultation teams in that there is a strong emphasis on dialectics. The DBT team emphasizes the same dialectic as DBT therapy: acceptance and change. And just as in DBT, this is not a dilution of either pole, nor a compromise, nor a 50:50 balance. This means holding both poles, acceptance and change, in their full intensity throughout the team: deep validation, understanding, and phenomenological empathy for teammates and clients are essential in team, as is the strong emphasis on continuously improving and enhancing the effectiveness of the therapy provided. This means not only discussing what interventions to provide to clients, but pushing the team member to provide more precise, scientifically driven, generally better DBT, addressing obstacles to adherent treatment, while simultaneously providing the emotional support, validation, and caring needed to do so.

Teammates may intervene with validation or change strategies as needed, while emphasizing the importance of both throughout the team. Team members need to feel cared for, understood, and supported, while at the same time given the (at times tough) feedback that they may need to do something differently. For certain teammates, being corrected and challenged decreases motivation, so the team must find a delicate balance where there is a strong push for change, along with a strong sense of support and acceptance. And once again, while the team holds both of these poles as essential, they intervene with exactly what is needed in any given moment. For example, a team member may only need validation: "I already have a solution, but I am still feeling really frustrated with one particular client. Can you validate the frustration?" The team may want to confirm that the solution is effective, but most of the time in team will then be spent on validating the member and reinforcing the effective strategies already implemented. Alternatively, a provider may want very little validation and a lot of practical help: "Let's not spend any time on validating me, I just need a solution and fast!" In either case, teams remain dialectical, holding both poles as fully important in every team meeting. There are other important dialectics that may also arise in team; teammates focus on finding the validity in both poles, searching for what is left out, and striving for synthesis.

The Culture of DBT Teams

To support DBT teams and the elements that make DBT unique from other types of consultation teams, we now discuss how to develop and maintain a DBT team culture, or set of shared goals and practices, to enhance the team's functioning and each member's ability to provide effective DBT. DBT team culture focuses on the elements described above, with an overarching emphasis on acceptance and change. In order to achieve this goal, there are a number of practices DBT teams implement, including team agreements, assumptions about clients and therapy, team roles, and a team agenda, which bring the team together around a similar perspective and value system. It will be important to avoid becoming rigid about these agreements and practices. They are guidelines that are designed to help the team function well, and while the team will benefit from attending to them regularly, it may at times be more effective to ignore certain problems, or delay dealing with them, depending on the team's priorities at any given time. The team can discuss at times whether not attending to certain problems is effective and helpful, or if it is ineffective (e.g., due to avoidance of conflict or emotion).

Core DBT Team Agreements

First, to help maintain the culture in the team, DBT team members agree to follow DBT team agreements.* The core agreements were originally described in Linehan (1993, pp. 117–119). These agreements are widely used in DBT teams (see Handout 1). They can help provide the backbone to the team's culture; they form the principles for team functioning.

1. *Dialectical Agreement.* The DBT team agrees to accept, at least pragmatically, a dialectical philosophy. There is no absolute truth; therefore, when polarities arise, the task is to search for the synthesis rather than for the truth. The dialectical agreement does not proscribe strong opinions, nor does it suggest that polarities are undesirable. Rather, it simply points to the direction team members agree to take when passionately held polar positions threaten to divide the team.

2. *Consultation-to-the-Client Agreement.* The DBT team agrees that team members do not serve as intermediaries for clients with other professionals, including other members of the team. The team agrees that clients will have more opportunity to learn when a DBT provider consults with clients on how to interact with other team members. When providers intervene on behalf of clients, clients lose that opportunity to learn to resolve problems themselves. Thus, when a clinician says things that are unhelpful or ineffective to the client, the task of the other team members is to help their clients cope with this provider's behavior, not necessarily to reform the provider. This does not mean that the team members do not conduct therapy for the therapist, plan treatment for their clients together, exchange information about the clients (including their problems with other members of the team), and discuss problems in treatment. DBT providers strive to provide such learning opportunities, and only intervene on behalf of clients when it is effective to do so.

3. *Consistency Agreement.* Failures in carrying out treatment plans can be problematic; at the same time, they present opportunities for

---

*Adapted from Linehan (1993, pp. 117–119). Copyright © 1993 The Guilford Press. Adapted by permission.

clients to learn to deal with the real world. The job of the DBT team is not to provide a stress-free, perfect environment for clients. Thus, the DBT team, including all members of the team, agrees that consistency of team members with one another is not necessarily expected; each member does not have to teach the same thing, nor do all have to agree on what are "proper rules" for therapy. Team members can each make their own decisions about how to proceed in therapy, within the DBT frame. Similarly, although it can make for smooth sailing when all members of an institution, agency, or clinic communicate the rules accurately and clearly, mix-ups are viewed as inevitable and isomorphic with the world we all live in. Any time a team member, team, or agency delivers treatment inconsistently (both in relation to other providers and to themselves), it is seen as a chance for clients (as well as team members) to practice the skills taught in DBT.

4. *Observing-Limits Agreement.* The team agrees that all members are to observe their own personal and professional limits. Furthermore, team members agree not to judge limits different from their own as too narrow or too broad, and instead determine if the limits are effective in a given situation. The team may suggest that a member broaden or narrow limits to become more effective, and at the same time will accept each other's differing limits without judgment. Team members will do their best to communicate their limits effectively to clients and teammates, and at the same time, clients are expected to ask about, learn, and accept providers' limits.

5. *Phenomenological Empathy Agreement.* DBT team members agree, all other things being equal, to search for nonpejorative or phenomenologically empathic interpretations of clients' behavior. The agreement is based on the fundamental assumption that clients are trying their best and want to improve, rather than to sabotage the therapy or "play games" with their provider. When a teammate is unable to come up with such an interpretation, other team members agree to assist in doing so, meanwhile also validating any frustration or other emotions that may arise for the provider. Thus, DBT team members agree to hold one another nonjudgmentally in the DBT frame. They agree to also search for a nonpejorative interpretation of the behavior of teammates, clients' family members, and any other relevant individuals, as well.

6. *Fallibility Agreement.* There is an explicit agreement in DBT teams that all team members are fallible. Thus, there is little need to be defensive, since it is agreed ahead of time that team members have

e whatever problematic things they are accused of doing. the team is to apply DBT principles to one another, in order ch member stay within DBT. As with clients, however, prob- ing with team members must be balanced with validation of the at wisdom of their stances. Because, in principle, all team members a allible, it is agreed that they will inevitably violate all of the agreements discussed here. When this is done, they will rely on one another to point out the polarity and will move on to search for the synthesis.

To these original core agreements, there are several additional agreements that we have found help teams to function well* (see Handout 2). These additions summarize the other practices typical to DBT teams, incorporating observer tasks and other strategies and guidelines most teams utilize to help maintain the team culture. These are outlined here and addressed in more detail throughout the book.

7. Consider oneself part of a community of therapists treating a community of clients. This means each teammate's clients are everyone's clients, and it is each person's responsibility to say something if a teammate has veered away from effective treatment.

8. Provide "therapy for the therapist" in the team; address each member's own and others' obstacles to providing DBT with fidelity to the manual. This means embodying DBT philosophy and strategies in team, including both acceptance and change, with oneself and each other. In other words, team members create an environment rich in validation, warmth, and acceptance, while at the same time giving feedback and addressing one's own and others' obstacles to providing DBT with fidelity to the manual. This is a commitment to search for what is valid in each teammate's experience even when it is difficult to do so, and to give feedback even when it is difficult to do so (e.g., when a teammate has more experience, or might get upset, or is another team member's boss, or is not sure about being "right"). Team members are vulnerable, share mistakes, and experience and express emotion in team; they accept validation and change-focused feedback. There is also a commitment to maintaining the confidentiality of any information disclosed in the team meeting, just as one would for a therapy session.

---

* Adapted with permission from Marsha M. Linehan, unpublished, University of Washington Behavioral Research and Therapy Clinics.

9. Provide DBT; not combine, alternate between, or : treatment modalities unless doing so effectively and mind: DBT one might add another cognitive-behavioral therapy ual while treating quality-of-life-interfering targets such : compulsive disorder [OCD] or binge eating). This allows for a common language and conceptualization of the treatment.

10. Conceptualize clients' and each other's behavior from a behavioral perspective; do not combine or add in other theoretical models. Many providers prefer eclecticism rather than a single theoretical approach. In DBT, maintaining a consistent, single, comprehensive philosophical approach with compatible theories is essential to inform the conceptualization of client and provider behaviors and related treatment decisions. The overarching theory for DBT and the DBT team is behaviorism, which will be discussed extensively in this book. Dialectics, biosocial theory, Zen practice, acceptance strategies, and change strategies are all viewed through a behavioral lens. Changing theories within a client's treatment (e.g., from behavioral to psychodynamic and back again) can lead to less precise explanations for behavior and therefore less leverage when generating solutions. Again, consistency allows the team to speak in the same language, communicate clearly, and approach the intervention from the same perspective.

11. Treat team meetings as importantly as any other therapy session; that is, attend weekly as often as possible, do not double schedule, arrive on time, stay until the end, come to meetings adequately prepared, speak in every team meeting (although not everyone needs to be on the agenda in every team), and participate in team by sharing the roles of meeting leader, observer, and/or any other roles essential to the team.

12. Be available to fulfill the role for which one joined the team (e.g., individual therapist, skills trainer, pharmacotherapist); all members of the DBT team have client contact and clinical responsibility. If one takes a break from seeing clients, one would also take a break from attending team.

13. Be willing to call out the "elephant in the room" when others do not. Each member will work to address unspoken "elephants," including speaking up if team is frustrating or not useful, broaching topics even when afraid of another team member's response, and not treating each other or oneself as too fragile to handle the discussion. This does not mean addressing every single problem in team; it emphasizes the

importance of communicating directly about problems interfering with providing DBT or with effective team functioning, when it is effective to do so.

14. Remain one-mindful in team, rather than doing two things at once; for example, do not attend to phone calls, texts, notes, or other distractions during team, nor engage in side conversations in team.

15. Assess sufficiently before offering solutions.

16. Strive to follow the assumptions about clients (Linehan, 1993) and therapy (see "DBT Assumptions" below).

17. Follow team policy regarding providing coverage for each other, missing team, and missing appointments with clients.

18. Continue focusing on all of the above, even when feeling burned out, frustrated, tired, overworked, underappreciated, hopeless, ineffective, etc.

DBT Assumptions about Clients*

In addition to these agreements, DBT team members choose to adhere to a set of assumptions about their clients and the therapy (see Handout 3). Adopting these assumptions affects how one thinks about the team's clients and their treatment and are therefore an integral part of the culture of the DBT team. These are assumptions, not facts; they cannot be proven "true" or "false"; rather they are a set of assumptions DBT team members *choose* to believe in to make their work more effective.

1. *Clients are doing the best they can.* It can be very tempting to believe clients are not trying, particularly when they engage in behavior that is frustrating to the provider or harmful to the treatment. Returning to this assumption can reduce team members' frustration and burnout. The team can help each team member maintain this stance, even in the face of very difficult behaviors. The team can provide reminders that even though the client was capable of engaging in this new, more skillful behavior last week, the client could not this week.

2. *Clients want to improve.* This is closely related to the first assumption. This assumption means that when a client is not improving, it is

---

*See Linehan (1993) for a full description.

due to emotion, lack of skill, cognitions, learning history, and other factors that are interfering with improving the client's life. The team can remind each member that it is more effective to believe the client wants to improve, and that there are factors interfering with such improvement. The team can also facilitate assessment and effective intervention when improvement is not occurring.

3. *Clients need to do better, try harder, and be more motivated to change.* This may seem to contradict the first two assumptions, but in actuality both poles are true. While clients may be doing the best they can and want to improve, it is typically the case that their current efforts are not sufficient to change their lives. It is each provider's job to analyze and understand the obstacles to the client making progress; in turn, it is the team's job to help the team member assess those obstacles and facilitate solutions.

4. *Clients may not have caused all of their own problems, but they have to solve them anyway.* This assumption highlights the fact that it is the clients themselves who will have to solve their problems, even if they did not create them. While it is true that clients do not know how to solve their problems on their own (or they would not need DBT!), expecting a provider or the world to take care of clients' problems for them will not provide a long-term solution to the client's problems. The team can help each member stick to this assumption by balancing working hard for clients while encouraging clients to also work hard to solve problems themselves.

5. *The lives of our clients can be unbearable.* It can be tempting, when a client does not engage in therapy as fully as we wish, to assume the client simply does not want to change. This assumption reminds everyone in team that the client is suffering, and there are obstacles interfering with change that can be solved once they are identified.

6. *Clients must learn new behaviors in all relevant contexts.* Clients will need to learn new skills and ways of coping in all possible settings (including contexts outside the therapy room), as well as across different emotional contexts they may experience. Helping the client tolerate stress without ineffective escape (e.g., effectively making it through a crisis instead of getting hospitalized, taking drugs, or using other escape strategies) requires a great deal of skill on the provider's part. This may require phone contact, structural changes in the environment, and other interventions that help clients learn to change not just in the therapy

room, but in their own environment. Because this can lead to more time spent on client care outside of session, as well as more opportunities to inadvertently reinforce ineffective behavior, and possibly more burnout for the provider, the team is essential in helping balance the client's needs with the provider's limits, in order to provide the best care.

7. *Clients cannot fail in therapy.* When clients do not progress or improve, or they leave therapy before meeting their goals, this assumption states that either the treatment was not sufficient for them or the provider did not apply the treatment as it was designed to be delivered. In DBT, a client's lack of progress is not considered the client's "fault." This assumption can be quite emotional for team members; it often feels as though the client simply does not step up to the plate to make the necessary changes, which can be frustrating and disappointing. Providers themselves can also feel blamed by this assumption, as if the client's lack of engagement is *their* fault. The purpose of this assumption is not to blame any member of the team; it is actually to remove blame altogether. Blame and judgment cloud our ability to assess and determine where the problem lies. For example, if I assume my client "just doesn't want to change," I stop assessing, and I don't realize that there is significant reinforcement for staying the same, and little reinforcement for changing certain behaviors. And by missing that information, I will feel frustrated with my client instead of solving the contingency management problem. The best any DBT provider can do is to follow the manual and provide treatment to fidelity. Assuming the provider follows the manual, and the team helps to hold the provider to the manual, when the treatment does not work it is because the treatment is insufficient for the client. No treatment works for everyone, and our understanding of human behavior is limited. We do not have solutions for every person and problem. It may be that that we simply do not know how to get a particular client to engage in treatment, or how to keep certain clients alive. That is a failure of the treatment and of the state of our science, not of the client, nor of the provider. It is also important to remember that "fail" has no moral judgment attached to it, it simply means "it did not work," that the goals were not attained. The team can monitor the culture of the team to ensure that such blame does not surface, and the focus remains on solid assessment and the provision of the most effective treatment possible.

8. *DBT team members need support.* This assumption forms the backbone of this book. DBT providers will make mistakes, and many

times those mistakes can interfere with the client's progress. DBT providers, just like our clients, will get pulled toward actions that reduce distress in the short run, but are not always effective in the long run. Clients will inadvertently shape providers toward ineffective choices at times. Even at their most skillful, team members need emotional support to provide effective DBT. Working in isolation, a provider can drift far from the manual, and face burnout and other difficulties. As we will discuss throughout this book, the primary functions of the DBT team are to continuously help each member to come back to the best care possible, as well as to maintain sufficient motivation to engage in this difficult work.

DBT Assumptions about Therapy*

1. *The most caring thing a DBT provider can do is help clients change in ways that bring them closer to their own ultimate goals.* This means the provider may push for change even when it is difficult for the client (e.g., continuing with exposure even when it is aversive) or slow down the push for change because to do so is deemed more effective for the client's care. The team will focus on this as its main goal: to help the team member effectively move clients toward their goals. If the team notices the team member has been shaped out of targeting certain behaviors, the team will highlight this problem, even if it is uncomfortable or difficult. With respect to the team, this might be restated to read, "The most caring thing a team can do is help its team members help clients change in ways that bring them closer to their own ultimate goals."

2. *Clarity, precision, and compassion are of the utmost importance in the conduct of therapy.* This means that not only is a provider warm and supportive, but also has precise, strategic interventions whenever possible, with a clear conceptualization, treatment plan, and rationale for each move in therapy. For example, a provider validating for an entire therapy session may be seen as compassionate but not helpful; however, if the provider mindfully chooses to avoid requesting change for a strategic reason for one full session, this choice could be considered effective DBT. We have seen many DBT providers emphasize clarity and precision over compassion and vice versa; team members often need help to synthesize

---

*Adapted with permission from Marsha M. Linehan, unpublished, University of Washington Behavioral Research and Therapy Clinics.

the two poles. The team can help maintain the balance with its focus on building empathy for the client as well as helping the clinician provide the most precise, clear interventions and strategies possible. The team can also help maintain this balance in team, when providing therapy for the therapist.

3. *The therapeutic relationship is a real relationship between equals.*

4. *Principles of behavior are universal, affecting DBT providers no less than clients.* The assumption of equality often creates an emotional reaction for DBT providers. Assumptions 3 and 4 assume that we, provider and client, are equal in that we are both susceptible to the principles of behaviorism, we both can be shaped toward effective and ineffective behaviors, and we are both a product of our biology and our environment. This is not to ignore the inherent power differential in the provider–client relationship; this discrepancy exists because the provider was fortunate enough to learn skills and interventions, and perhaps was born with a different biology than the client, and therefore has certain knowledge and abilities that the client does not possess. The team can monitor when members drift from this assumption, and help them return to the notion that the client is operating within the same principles as the provider, and in that respect, they are indeed equals. This can increase the team member's compassion and ability to conceptualize a case skillfully.

5. *DBT providers can fail.* This is yet another provocative assumption for many DBT providers. When we teach this to DBT providers, many start worrying about suicide and lawsuits if they are unable to perform perfectly all of the time, a high bar indeed! The idea of failing is highly charged for most of us. DBT does not, however, expect or require providers to be perfect. As mentioned in the assumptions about clients, if we can define the term "fail" in nonjudgmental terms, meaning simply that the goal was not reached (in this case, the manual was not followed exactly), this assumption can be easier to grasp. Any DBT provider can *fail* to provide the treatment as it is described in the treatment manual; this is actually expected, given the many obstacles that may arise. This is considered so typical, in fact, that this was one of the primary reasons the DBT team was developed. The team helps the team member identify, assess, and intervene each time the member stops doing DBT. This is a failure in the sense that the treatment was not provided as designed,

as opposed to a reflection on anyone's capability or character, or any sense of "fault." It is simply a statement of fact. The team participates by acknowledging that this is true, and being willing to identify it when they see it, in order to help each member tolerate the inevitable emotion and turn back toward the treatment if drift has occurred.

6. *The treatment can fail even when DBT providers do not.* The team can also remind each member that just because a treatment is not working does not mean the provider has failed to do something. Just as chemotherapy does not always work for cancer patients, our best interventions do not always work, even when delivered with fidelity. As described previously, the state of the science of behavior change is limited; if a DBT provider is utilizing the manual and the team, the most likely obstacle is that we do not have ideal interventions for all of our clients. The team can lend support around this assumption, as well as offer suggestions for when it might be time to stop the treatment or change strategies.

Other Elements of Team Structure

Along with these agreements and assumptions, DBT teams use roles and an agenda to help maintain the structure and culture of DBT. The roles of team leader, meeting leader, and observer are most common in DBT teams, but some teams also add additional roles to help maintain the structure and culture of the team.

The elements discussed here, including team functions, agreements, assumptions, and structure, together create the heart of the team. While this may seem like an extensive amount of structure, these principles are pulled directly from DBT treatment, and will likely be familiar to DBT providers.

Starting with the foundation of these principles and strategies, teams may need to adapt this structure to meet their specific needs. When teams notice the urge to adapt or eliminate one of these elements, it will be important to consider the dialectic: the validity of the original structure and the validity of the desire to alter it. Considering both of these poles will help teams avoid taking the path of least resistance (e.g., eliminating an agreement because it is difficult to follow or because the team wishes to avoid conflict), and maximize the chances the team will design a structure that is most beneficial to the team, team members, and clients. Teams can remain alert to urges to change the structure: while flexibility is essential, changing spontaneously may lead to emotion-mind decisions. It is helpful to be flexible and strategic when deciding these elements, then to follow them carefully even when it is challenging to do so. Instead of changing elements when following them feels difficult, teams will likely benefit from reviewing and revising them on a regular basis, such as at an annual retreat.

Teams may also want to add structure; for example, a team full of trainees may need to focus more on teaching and modeling during team; a research team may need to add an emphasis on a specific treatment target or on following a particular research protocol. Teams in inpatient or residential settings may need to address the difficulty of working different shifts; while the individual therapist remains the primary provider, these teams may need to create systems to maintain effective communication across multiple staff, such as adding additional meetings, engaging in structured communication and/or occasional formal team meetings with swing and night shift, and creating means to inform the individual therapist of developments in the client's care. Teams may also need to develop strategies for communicating if they are meeting via video conference.

Providers who do not use DBT may also wish to develop a treatment team with similar goals and structure. We are aware of other treatments that use a team approach for treatments other than DBT (e.g., CBT for anxiety); mentalization-based treatment for BPD (Bateman & Fonagy, 2004): treatment for depressed and suicidal adolescents (Brent, Poling, & Goldstein, 2011); and trauma systems therapy (Saxe, Ellis, & Kaplow, 2007), suggesting providers of other treatments may benefit from the DBT team approach. Within the principles and structure discussed in this book, there are many ways to adjust the elements of the DBT team to fit the specific needs of a particular treatment, team members, and clients.

The Structure of This Book

Expanding upon the concepts introduced in this chapter, Chapter 2 describes the systems, roles, and tasks that help DBT teams function well. This includes the jobs the team will need to accomplish to run effectively, and how the meeting leader, observer, and other roles can help the team maintain the culture.

Chapter 3 focuses specifically on the role of team leader and the unique challenges inherent in that role. This chapter discusses how to guide a program and multiple team members, and associated difficulties that may accompany this role. Team leaders are also in a position of both leading and being a member of the treatment team simultaneously, which can present dilemmas that require particular attention and care.

Chapter 4 addresses the structure of DBT team meetings, and how to use an agenda to support an effective structure. This chapter includes a discussion of time management and prioritization in team meetings.

Chapter 5 goes into more depth on the concept of *therapy for the therapist,* and how team members can provide support and facilitate change for their teammates. This chapter includes DBT strategies and skills, and suggestions for ways teammates can implement them with each other, not just with their clients.

Chapter 6 describes several problems that are common in DBT teams, all of which can present obstacles to an effective team process. Means of assessing and understanding these problems are discussed along with suggestions for the resolution of such problems.

Chapter 7 focuses on one of the most challenging situations in team: when a client, a provider, and therefore a team experience a suicide crisis. The important roles teams play before, during, and after a suicide crisis are discussed.

And finally, Chapter 8 explains how to start a new DBT team, as well as how to bring new members onto a DBT team.

Each chapter ends with "Ideas for Practice," which provide suggestions for ways to practice the strategies or concepts in each chapter. These exercises are simply starting points for teams to create their own practices that are tailored to their own needs.

It is important to note that this is not intended to be a rule book or a lock-step manual. This book focuses on principles, not mandates, for dealing with a variety of situations flexibly and strategically, with examples and exercises that can be tailored to many teams. While we find the structure provided here is helpful in developing an effective team, there is no one "right" way to structure a team. The principles are much more important than the overt appearance of the team. Each team is so unique that its problems and solutions will vary widely. When teams become rigid or stuck on rules, while ignoring what is actually helpful to its members, clients, and the team as a whole, they typically run into trouble. We recommend starting as close to the traditional model as possible, learn what works and does not work, then mindfully and strategically adjust as needed, and monitor the effectiveness of those adjustments. The use of tailored application of these principles, as well as creativity and responsiveness to the individuals within each unique team, is emphasized throughout this book.

A Note on Language

We made every effort to use gender-neutral pronouns throughout the text. We relied on plural pronouns wherever possible and used "they" or "one" when a singular pronoun was required. The only exceptions (in which we used "he" and "she" as pronouns) were examples that referred to specific individuals.

Conclusion

DBT teams are considered an essential part of DBT, based on the premise that skillful DBT therapists are essential to delivering effective DBT. This chapter describes the purpose of the DBT team, including an overarching focus on fidelity to the DBT manuals, with an emphasis on enhancing the motivation and capability of the providers on the team. We describe the ways in which DBT teams are different from traditional consultation teams, and we introduce several components that support the culture of the DBT team, including agreements, assumptions, and other structural elements. We expand upon these concepts throughout this book. We hope that by providing these principles for DBT teams, we can help DBT providers create and maintain a community, a place where they find comfort, support, ideas, knowledge, and growth, from which they can provide the best DBT possible.

DBT Team Tasks and Roles
Who Does What?

D BT teams vary widely in their structure, in the number and type of providers attending, and in many other aspects. Across teams, certain tasks have emerged as important to most teams. The aim of these team tasks is to support fidelity to the DBT manual, maintain an effective culture in the team, and enhance provider capability and motivation. This chapter describes these tasks; however, it is important to note that each team has unique needs, and therefore each team can adjust these tasks to make sure they are fulfilling the overall team goals. These team components are deliberately not stated as rules, but rather as principles to be followed in a flexible manner. Some teams may handle these informally, or not need them at all; many larger teams will find formally addressing them will be helpful. The tasks we have found helpful across most teams include:

1. Managing time in team.
2. Alerting team members when behaviors deviate from the DBT manual and the team agreements.
3. Documenting decisions and suggestions made in team meetings.
4. Assigning and rotating roles within the team.
5. Addressing team member absences (both from team and from therapy sessions).

We have found that these functions can be met most easily when team members fulfill certain roles. Once again, teams may adapt or combine these roles and tasks, add to them, or choose not to use some of them at all. Continuous monitoring of the effectiveness of these strategies will ensure that these roles are used to their best advantage. Many teams, including ours, use the following roles to support the structure of the team and the overall fidelity of the treatment provided:*

- Team leader (discussed in Chapter 3)
- Meeting leader
  - Sets agenda.
  - Reminds team of core team agreements.
  - Manages time on the agenda.
  - Closes team meeting.
- Observer
  - Monitors DBT team discussions.
  - Alerts the team when team members deviate from the expanded list of team agreements.
  - Asks for change as needed.
- Notetaker
  - Documents team discussions.
  - Facilitates follow-through from team members.
- Role manager
  - Tracks the rotation of roles.
- Client coverage/team attendance manager
  - Creates and monitors a system for team attendance and absences.
  - Maintains policy for client coverage; creates a system for communicating about client coverage when team members are absent.
  - Monitors whether team members make their repair to team, and reminds them to do so when they forget.

For each of the above roles, we discuss the primary tasks and one or more ways to complete those tasks. As previously mentioned, teams have a great deal of flexibility in utilizing these roles. Meeting leader and observer are essential; the other tasks are important, but may be divided

---

* Adapted with permission from Marsha M. Linehan, unpublished, University of Washington Behavioral Research and Therapy Clinics.

among members or otherwise assigned, rather than having the specific roles of notetaker, role manager, and coverage/absence manager. Many teams have created additional roles, as well; teams can consider where their particular challenges lie and implement these as needed. Examples are discussed below. Teams typically rotate responsibility for many of these roles, most importantly meeting leader and observer, such that everyone has the experience of leading the team meeting and functioning as observer. Teams may choose how often the roles rotate; MML's team rotates once per month and JS's team rotates every week. One person may fulfill more than one role, as well. Because the role of team leader is discussed in Chapter 3, that role will not be expanded upon here.

Meeting Leader

The meeting leader manages how time is spent in team meetings. This role is distinct from that of the team leader. In contrast to the team leader, the meeting leader role can rotate regularly; it does not require a consistent person. The meeting leader sets and manages the agenda (described in detail in Chapter 4), then moves the team through the agenda, which focuses primarily on leading a mindfulness exercise or assigning another member to do so; reading one of the meeting leader's agreement reminders; asking the notetaker to read or display the last meeting's notes; and addressing the remaining topics on the agenda. The meeting leader makes sure essential items are covered and the team does not spend more time than planned on each agenda item. The meeting leader announces whose turn it is to speak, uses a clock or timer to monitor how much time is spent on each item, and alerts members when their turn is nearly up.

Setting the Agenda

There are a variety of ways the leader might set the agenda. Teams may verbally set their agenda at the start of the team meeting, with the leader quickly writing down the needs of the team members in the room. One of our (JS) teams uses an agenda form (see Chapter 4 for examples) that team members fill out as they enter the room, such that no time is spent discussing the agenda. The meeting leader can then use that form to structure time throughout the meeting. Our other (MML) team places the agenda on a whiteboard, with team members writing their requests where all team members can see them. An electronic agenda displayed by projector is yet another option. With any of these methods, the agenda provides the structure around which the meeting leader organizes team time.

Reminding the Team of the Core Team Agreements

The meeting leader also has the task of reminding the team of the core DBT team agreements (see Handout 1). I (MML) expanded upon these particular agreements in more detail because they are so central to the culture of the team. The meeting leader reminds the team by reading one core DBT team agreement, in full, at the start of each meeting. The meeting leader may choose any agreement. The principle is to keep these agreements salient in each team meeting to minimize drift. In brief, the core DBT team agreements are:

1. Dialectical Agreement
2. Consultation-to-the-Client Agreement
3. Consistency Agreement
4. Observing-Limits Agreement
5. Phenomenological Empathy Agreement
6. Fallibility Agreement

Typically, teams print the full text of these agreements and have it available in every team meeting. See Chapter 1 for a discussion of these agreements.

Managing Time on the Agenda

Teams also vary widely on how strictly they adhere to the timing of the agenda. With smaller teams, or teams with ample time, the meeting leader may not monitor time as closely. When teams are large or have a significant number of agenda items, however, the meeting leader can ask members to be very specific about how much time they would like, and then monitor the time closely such that each high-priority agenda item receives team time. Based on the priority given (prioritization is discussed further in Chapter 4), the meeting leader decides who speaks first, second, and so on, and alerts each team member when it is time to move on to the next agenda item.

Many teams have certain team members who are reluctant to stop talking, even once the requested time has expired. Often members will have a strong urge to make their points, even when there is no remaining time for that topic. In such a situation, the meeting leader highlights the problem and attempts to move the conversation to the next team member. If a team member is still reluctant to move on, this becomes a problem to solve: the leader, observer, or any other member may place the topic of time management on the agenda, or if the team agrees this provider's topic remains a very high priority, the meeting leader may ask other members to give up some of their time to allow a continuation of the current discussion.

Closing the Team Meeting

Finally, the meeting leader closes the team meeting at the appointed time. Depending on the culture and needs of the team, the ending may include ringing the bell, shifting the topic to the sharing of effective provider and/or client behaviors, or otherwise informing the team that the meeting has ended.

Observer

The observer's role supports the second task: to monitor the team discussions. This role brings the team's attention to moments when any member strays from the expanded list of DBT team agreements, or otherwise engages in behavior that may not be beneficial to the client, a team member, or the culture of the team (e.g., when the team gets polarized, or there is an elephant in the room that no one is addressing), and asks for effective change as needed.

The observer observes team discussions, keeping the Observer Reminders in view during the team meeting to pay special attention to a particular subset of the team agreements. Similar to the meeting leader, the observer uses this subset of the agreements to monitor ongoing team process and facilitate effective team functioning. This list reflects common examples of how a team might fall out of the DBT frame, as defined by one or more of the agreements. This is not an exhaustive list, but merely problems that come up frequently in the teams we have worked with. We have found this particular set of reminders most useful for the observer, but a team could add other agreements and additional behaviors in an effort to address particular team problems. See Handout 4 for a reproducible page the observer can use during team; we also included Handout 5, a checklist for observers to monitor how the team intervenes when these problems arise.

Observer Reminders* include:

1. A team member did not speak during team.
2. Nonmindfulness; a team member did two things at once.
3. A team member was late or unprepared.
4. A team member was defensive.
5. A team member made a judgmental or noncompassionate comment.
6. Solutions were offered before sufficient problem definition/assessment occurred.
7. A team member was treated as fragile; there was an elephant in the room that was not discussed.
8. A dialectic went unresolved.

For all of these reminders, the observer and the team can decide how the observer is to get the team's attention. In our teams, the observer rings a mindfulness singing bowl (or "bell") whenever one of these behaviors is noticed. In other teams, this has evolved into the observer simply saying, "Ring the bell" without actually ringing the bell; the statement is sufficient to get the team's attention. A team can use any means, with words, sounds, or gestures to notify other members.

The observer reminders are discussed in turn below.

1. *A team member did not speak during team.* When an individual does not speak for the duration of the team, it affects the rest of the team. Not speaking results in less disclosure, and therefore less vulnerability in team. Individuals may not speak for many reasons, including:

* Not being one-mindful
* Frustration with the team

---

*Adapted with permission from Marsha M. Linehan, unpublished, University of Washington Behavioral Research and Therapy Clinics.

- Lack of experience, or fear of not having the "right" thing to say, or the belief they do not know enough to be able to comment
- Exhaustion
- Hope that someone else will speak up first
- Not able to find a break in the conversation

Team members do not need to place themselves on the agenda every meeting, nor is it helpful to talk just for the sake of talking. In large teams, it may be particularly difficult to have a chance to speak often. The principle here is the importance of each member remaining actively engaged in the conversation and participating in validation, assessment, and solution generation for the other teammates. The observer can watch for team members' silence, assess if there is a problem (e.g., not speaking because someone else already said what they were going to say is not problematic; not speaking because someone is checked out or frustrated with the team could negatively impact the culture of the team), then move forward effectively.

When an observer notices a provider not speaking in team, the observer can decide whether an intervention is necessary; such interventions might include ringing the bell, saying, "You're quiet today, what's up?" assessing if there is an elephant in the room, directly asking for that person to weigh in on a particular topic, or any other way to highlight and/or rectify the situation.

2. *Nonmindfulness; a team member did two things at once; a lack of one-mindfulness during the team meeting.* This might include:

- Looking spaced out, not paying attention
- Checking one's phone, texting, e-mailing
- Having a side conversation
- Doing paperwork

When one commits to being on a team, one commits to being there fully. If any team members are not fully present, the observer or other members can alert them and ask them to return their attention to the team. The observer could give a number of responses, including saying in a light tone, "Hey, we aren't very mindful today! Let's try to focus!" or "I desperately need your attention, I have a problem!" or "Would you please put your phone away." or "Is something going on with one of your clients? I notice you are on your phone a lot today."

3. *A team member was late or unprepared for team.* The team agrees to place as much emphasis on the team meeting as it does on client meetings. In other words, other meetings or obligations do not trump team time. Phone calls, e-mail, getting lunch or coffee, or going to the dentist are all common reasons to miss team, but can make other team members feel less valued, deprive the team of that individual's contribution, and affect team morale. These absences also become part of the culture, such that the team may be faced with multiple absences on a regular basis.

Many teams require a chain and solution analysis from a late team member. Arriving late to team can result in team frustration and distraction, so it is often important to address. However, conducting the chain/solution analysis in team also results in lost time. Teams may find it helpful to have the absent member complete the chain outside of team, or quickly discuss in team, in order to maximize effective use of team time. There is dialectic here: on the one hand, spending time to assess and solve the tardiness together as a team is important; at the same time, the team may wish to save that time for providing therapy for the therapist. If the team member can solve the problem of tardiness without taking team time, that is the best option; if the tardiness continues, it affects the whole team and becomes a high priority for the team to address within the team meeting. The observer can help the team notice the tardiness and make sure solutions are identified as needed.

On the other hand, the team will likely not mind a teammate arriving a couple of minutes late once every several months, or missing a meeting on occasion for vacation. Just as with clients, if it is not causing harm in the team, the team may choose to ignore it or wait to determine if it is indeed a significant problem. Our teams ask members to text or e-mail the team in advance if they will be late or absent, and only assess/solve if the team member has an unplanned absence or a pattern of absences. A culture focused on very tight rules can decrease the enjoyment in team; the team can address this dialectic and choose at what point interventions might be needed, balancing the importance of attendance with the need for flexibility.

Arriving unprepared is another behavior that may frustrate the team. Examples include:

- Forgetting/failing to bring up client issues.
- Not remembering a client issue from several days prior.

- Not preparing for "team member of the week" (see p. 42).
- Otherwise not preparing to present consultation items.
- Not taking the time to eat/get food, use the restroom, etc., prior to the start of the meeting, in order to be fully one-mindful at the meeting.

It may take some preparation time to get one's needs met in team. Team members agree to set aside time in advance to be sure they are prepared and everyone can maximize their time in team. The observer can gently and/or irreverently remind team members of this agreement.

4. *A team member was defensive.* The observer will highlight when team members appear defensive in response to feedback from the team. For example, they:

- Are not open to team feedback, defend themselves instead of listening to what others are suggesting or highlighting.
- "Yeah, but . . . " or shoot down every suggestion, insisting they've already tried every suggestion given.
- Deny any fallibility (a nondialectical response), without considering there may be validity in the other pole.
- Agree overtly, and privately disagree with feedback; they have no commitment to consider or implement feedback.

When team members are more focused on protecting themselves or improving others' view of them than learning and benefiting from consultation, it can have a significant impact on the team's willingness to highlight and discuss problems with that particular team member. It is important that team members can disagree and openly examine both sides of clinical issues. If the team highlights one pole while a particular member insists their own pole is correct, the team will become polarized. Assessing and helping the team member hear the feedback will often open up a dialogue about the team's and clinician's interaction. For example, an observer could say lightly, "Oh no! Has our feedback made you feel defensive?!" or "I think defensiveness has entered the room!" and/or validate the challenges of receiving tough feedback.

Being nondefensive does not, of course, translate to becoming passive or losing one's own perspective. It only means remaining open to feedback and exploring others' views; the team member can then make a wise decision about how to proceed. The team cannot control what providers do in their sessions; the team's job is to provide feedback and

additional perspectives to consider. This agreement is focused on each
member remaining open to these alternative ideas, interpretations, and
recommendations.

The team may also misinterpret a teammate's clarification as defensiveness. If the team is not absorbing information from a member, and
that member repeatedly tries to explain, the team may assume this rep-
etition is defensiveness. In such a case, the observer can highlight the
problem and suggest the team slow down and listen to the provider (as
opposed to addressing what appears to be defensiveness).

5. *A team member made judgmental or noncompassionate comments,*
including comments regarding:

- Clients
- Clients' family members (parents, spouse, etc.)
- Team members
- A school, government program, or other entity related to the
  client's situation
- A provider's own behavior or character
- The agency's administration

Again, the team members agree that maintaining a compassionate stance is essential, in order to remain helpful to the client, obtain
accurate data about the situation, and avoid burnout. When a teammate
is experiencing strong frustration about a situation, judgments can be
highly tempting. Judging can also be very subtle and easy to miss. The
observer monitors closely, and when noticed, highlights the judgment
and reminds the team about the DBT team agreements.

Teams might also mislabel a statement as a judgment. Opinions,
doubts, emotions, or worries are not necessarily judgments, as long as they
are not treated as facts. For example, "You shouldn't use that strategy with
your client," is a judgment; the "should" implies there is a "right" and a
"wrong" way to move forward. Instead, one could say, "I am worried that
this strategy will invalidate your client, and I'd like to continue brainstorming solutions that are more validating." The more clear and precise
team members can be in describing, the less likely judgments will arise.

Team members judging themselves is an important problem to
address in team, as well. The judgments lead to a loss of information
about the problem, as they point to an inaccurate explanation (e.g., "I'm
stupid" inhibits the identification of the actual controlling variables).
Judging oneself can have a strong impact on morale and limit understanding of the problem.

Self-judgments might include:

- Saying they "should" have known better, handled it differently, etc.
- Trying to stop an emotion using willpower (e.g., "I just need to stop reacting this way," or "I'm overreacting, I've got to pull myself together!")
- Insulting, degrading, or otherwise judging oneself for experiencing an emotion or engaging in other reactions to a clinical situation
- Judging oneself for not knowing the answer or the best way to move forward

Judgments can take many forms. The observer can monitor for any statements that may be judgmental or noncompassionate and simply inform or ask the team if there was a judgment made. An observer might simply ring the bell, or say, "I think that was a judgment!" or suggest the team member start the description over without judgments. The team member or the team as a whole can then decide if highlighting was sufficient, or if more time is needed to address the judgment.

While attending to judgments is important in maintaining DBT team culture, there will also be times when it is effective to let the judgment slide, or to wait a period of time before asking for a restatement. When a team member is very emotional, or makes an offhand comment (such as "I can't believe I did that, what an idiot!"), it may be helpful to focus on the judgments; it may also be helpful to focus on the problem at hand, and return to the judgments later if needed. Again, teams can guard against rigidity, use clinical and interpersonal skill with each other, and focus on effectiveness rather than perfection.

6. *Solutions were offered before sufficient problem definition/assessment occurred.* One of the main sources of frustration in team can come from teammates throwing out solutions before they understand the problem. This can result in the team spending significant time off-track and the team member who is asking for help feeling overwhelmed or misunderstood. The provider, observer, or any other member can alert the team when any of the following occur:

- The team immediately begins offering multiple solutions.
- It becomes clear the team does not know what the problem actually is.
- The team is not responding to the provider's request.
- The team's solutions are disorganized or unfocused.

It can be incredibly frustrating for everyone involved when the team offers solutions that have already been tried, or if the team is solving a different problem than the one placed on the agenda. Ensuring the team is focused on the right problem and has enough detail to aim the solutions at an effective component of the problem is essential. When it becomes clear that the team has prematurely moved to problem solving, the observer can alert the team that more assessment is required by saying, "Can we hang on for a second? I think you said you needed help with assessment, and we are offering solutions. Am I right about that?" or "If we can pause here, I'm not sure I even know what the problem is. Before we give more solutions, let's assess further."

There may be times when the team identifies problems other than the one the provider placed on the agenda. In such cases, the team can say, "Let's definitely talk through what you're struggling with. I'd also like to make a few comments about your treatment plan, so let's save a few minutes for that, too."

7. *A team member was treated as "fragile," there was an elephant in the room,* and the team held back on giving feedback or avoided speaking about a specific issue. Examples include:

- There is an important topic or emotion that is evident but not discussed.
- A member has an urge to say something important but does not, for fear of the reaction from the team or a particular member.
- There is tension between members and no one identifies it.

It is important not to "fragilize" team members, or assume they (or oneself!) are too fragile to handle a difficult conversation. In order for the team to thrive, there must be permission and encouragement to bring up difficult topics nonjudgmentally and talk them through. If team members avoid bringing up certain topics with a teammate, the problem will continue, the provider may drift from the treatment model and likely provide ineffective therapy, and the team culture may be negatively impacted. Team members may simultaneously validate the individual and consider that perspective while requesting a change in behavior (upholding the dialectic of acceptance and change).

This agreement does not suggest one be so confrontational that a teammate cannot digest the feedback. Presenting feedback too forcefully can be just as problematic as avoiding the feedback. This agreement simply means the team agrees to engage in the difficult conversations necessary to maximize the chances of effective treatment. Whether warm or irreverent, remaining descriptive, specific, and nonjudgmental is absolutely essential. Examples of comments that may be too forceful for some teammates include, "I can't believe you did that!" (which is judgmental as well as very forceful); "You aren't hearing anything the team is saying!"; or "You've got to change what you're doing or your client will die!" (At the same time, there may be moments when such strong language is needed to capture a teammate's attention.) Removing all judgment will help the team remain precise and on topic. Teams can strive to strike a balance between being nonjudgmentally direct, while also being mindful of ensuring the feedback is delivered in a way that can be heard and absorbed. An example of direct, nonjudgmental feedback might be, "I can totally see why you said that to your client. However, I think it might reinforce suicidality. Can we explore that possibility?" Effective communication will depend upon the teammate's style, team culture, level of trust in the team, and many other factors.

Orienting new team members ahead of time will also help providers adjust to the more direct communication in a DBT team. For some team members, shaping may be necessary. A person may agree to work on being more direct and receiving feedback more effectively, but that does not mean that all the right skills are in place. (Even highly skilled DBT providers may not want to be hit by feedback that feels like a Mack truck!) Some teams choose to throw a new teammate into the deep end by making very direct, forceful comments right away; this may work, but similar to other forms of flooding, may result in a quick departure from the team or lasting resentment. Each team can find a balance that is effective for the overall team, the individuals involved, and the particular situation.

8. *A dialectic went unresolved.* Many dialectics show up in any DBT team meeting. The team can become polarized on points such as the client needs to change immediately versus the client is already doing the best they can; or the client should end treatment versus the client should continue in DBT; or the provider should do more versus the provider should stop working harder than the client. The team may fall on two poles, or the team may unite on one pole and miss the validity in other perspectives. The concept of dialectics allows the team to hold two poles true at the same time, which creates a new context from which to

validate and solve problems. For example, if the team can state that the client is trying very hard, *and* they need to do more in order to reach their goals, this moves the team member and team out of a debate and into a dialectical stance. The potential for polarization, or for failing to hold both poles as true and instead trying to determine which pole is *right,* is nearly constant in team. The observer and the team at large must remain very aware of these moments and help the team become more dialectical. The observer might alert the team, "I think there's a dialectic here!" or "Can anyone bring up the other pole so we can stay dialectical?"

Flexiblity and mindfulness are important when observing the team: if an observer stops the team every single time someone is not perfectly following the DBT model, the team will not function, and everyone will be miserable! The observer can decide whether it is effective to let certain behaviors slide, or to wait until a pattern is clear before mentioning it, or to address each instance. For example, a teammate may appear checked-out for a minute in team; the observer may just watch and see if it is a chronic problem, and not address it if it is brief and has no impact on the team. Or when the observer notices a member of the team making judgmental statements, the observer might call attention to the judgment in order to remind the team of the team agreements, and/or request the team member to repeat the behavior in a more effective manner (e.g., restate the comment without the judgment). There will be times when the current discussion is more important than correcting a team member; the observer and other team members can decide when an intervention may not be necessary. The observer can also keep in mind the development of each provider; oftentimes the individual is making significant progress in becoming less judgmental or in arriving on time, and shaping progress will be more effective than demanding perfection.

There is also great flexibility with respect to the content of the observer reminders. Teams can add in other agreements or additional behaviors that will help team members remember to target certain changes or address components of team culture. For example, our (JS) team struggled at one point with trainees feeling reluctant to speak when very senior clinicians were on the team, and senior clinicians ended up talking much more than other members of the team. So the team expanded on the item focused on all team members speaking, to remind the observer to monitor comments made by trainees and senior clinicians. Our new observer reminder focused on getting those with less experience to talk more often, such that new members were taken seriously and had the opportunity to receive shaping and correction as needed. At another point we wanted to focus on putting the team member on the agenda more regularly, so we added, "The provider put the client on the agenda instead of themselves" to the reminders. The observer reminders are an opportunity to discuss and structure change in a team; tailored reminders can help the observer and the entire team to be mindful of specific team goals in addition to the general culture of the team.

Observer reminders can also lose their salience, and the team can become desensitized to the content of the observer reminders. In such a situation, the items no longer impact the behavior of the group and members no longer strive to change their own and others' behavior in team meetings. The observer may stop providing reminders, or the team may superficially say, "That was a judgment," but not actually attempt to change each other's judgmental language. Remaining aware of this likelihood may be quite helpful; we have also found that reviewing the reminders as a team on a regular basis, changing the language of the items, adding items to adapt to a team's changing needs, and otherwise engaging with the list mindfully can renew the interest in and dedication to these agreements. For example, a team could use 15 minutes of team time once every 3–4 months to review the observer reminders and discuss whether any additions are needed to fit the team's needs, or the team could make this an agenda item at an annual retreat.

Another difficulty is the observer's feedback can become aversive to team members, such that they have a strong negative response to the observer's comments. Team members may become defensive, roll their eyes, ignore the observer, continue with the original problematic behavior, and so on. There may be many sources of this problem; many teams identify the problem is that the observer's feedback is judgmental, or that a team member is not receiving sufficient validation, resulting in team tension. Assessing the problem before determining solutions will likely enhance the team's effectiveness at resolving this difficulty. See Chapter 6 for a discussion of this problem.

Notetaker

The notetaker documents the topics discussed in team. The purpose of these notes is to provide continuity from one team to the next; the notes can serve as a reminder to team members to return to the previous week's agenda items if needed, to tell the team the solutions were helpful, or ask for more help, or block any avoidance. If the provider cannot remember the previously provided suggestions, the notes provide a helpful reminder. Given that this is a community of therapists treating a community of clients, the notes also provide a helpful reminder to the rest of the team regarding progress with particular difficulties. Teams may prefer to make this a rotating role; it can be difficult to fully participate and take notes at the same time, and rotating this task can lessen the burden on any one particular provider. This role is optional; in some teams providers track their own commitment and follow-through on assignments from the team. This may be simpler, but runs the risk that the team may be less aware of a teammate's avoidance or other difficulties with follow-through. The team can discuss whether a notetaker would be a helpful addition.

When documenting therapy notes, the content can be minimal; the team can decide how much information is helpful to facilitate continuity. In our (JS) team, we document minimal details, tracking only the items that require follow-up in future teams. Other teams may choose to track team discussions in a more detailed fashion. See Handouts 6 (simplest documentation) and 7 (more detailed documentation) for sample formats. The notes typically include:

1. The agenda item or problem (keeping the focus on the provider).
2. Ideas and suggestions from the team.
3. Any specific steps a team member agrees to take with respect to implementing the solution (if relevant).

The notes are saved in a secure location. The notetaker then makes sure the notes are reviewed in the subsequent team meeting, and any ongoing topics are addressed.

The notes reflect DBT principles just as much as the team's conversations do. For example, the notetaker strives to be behaviorally specific and descriptive, using nonjudgmental language.

We are often asked whether these notes present protection or liability in terms of legal situations. It is not clear if team notes can offer additional protection in terms of legal liability. Documenting that one sought consultation can be helpful to demonstrate a provider is proceeding in a thoughtful manner, and showing attendance at a DBT team can also help demonstrate one is delivering an evidence-based treatment. While both of these should be helpful theoretically, such legal situations are so rare it is difficult to know whether these factors are essential.

We know of no teams that have been compelled to submit team notes for any legal situation. Liability and legal protection are concerns; at the same time, fear of legal liability can lead providers to make very ineffective decisions. We cannot provide any legal advice; however, we do recommend staying focused on following the DBT principles and manuals, in order to provide the most effective therapy possible, rather than making decisions about notes based on fear.

To enhance a sense of privacy with team notes, I (MML) sought consultation about whether team notes could be considered "therapy notes," meaning they could have the same confidentiality and privacy as our clients' medical records. One suggestion I received was to have teammates sign a confidentiality agreement, which could possibly increase the likelihood team notes would be considered the provider's own therapy notes (as opposed to notes about clients). We have included an example of such a confidentiality agreement (Handout 8), with the caution that there are circumstances (e.g., a court order) when any records may be required, even with the presence of such an agreement. Teammates should contact their malpractice carrier or attorney regarding such concerns, as we are unable to advise on legal matters.

Because these notes are for team members, not clients, if one believes it will be important to document team consultation regarding a particular client, we recommend the provider place a note directly in the client's chart. The team notes are not typically considered a formal part of a client's medical record, so the occurrence of consultation will not be officially documented unless the provider generates a specific note in that client's medical record regarding the team's consultation. For example, one might document, "Consulted with the DBT team on (date). Agreed to the following plan: . . . ." The provider should then document compliance with that particular plan.

Additionally, it is important that the notetaker avoids documenting suggestions as mandates or requirements. Giving team members mandates does not fit with the spirit of DBT team, where each member requests and receives consultation. In DBT, the individual therapist and client together are the "hub of the wheel," who direct the course of treatment, and the team's job is only to highlight problems and provide suggestions. While the team may be very direct in working to change any provider's course of action, the team does not give commands regarding any client's treatment. The phrasing of the notes should reflect the stance that providers receive ideas as suggestions, not mandates, and document the behaviors the team member agrees to engage in. (Of course, if one member is the supervisor or employer of another team member, there may be requirements for certain behaviors such as conducting risk assessments, particularly if one is working under the license of another team member. Agency policy, research protocols, licensing requirements, laws, and ethical codes may also create requirements for team members' behavior (e.g., paperwork, particular assessments, responses to high-risk situations, etc.). These requirements should be clearly outlined prior to engaging in clinical work together.

Role Manager

The role manager fulfills the fourth team function. This individual will assign and post the team roles in advance, in order to avoid spending team time determining who will fulfill which role. Once again, this role may not be needed in every team. Smaller teams in particular may have no need for this function, but larger teams may find the structure and organization helpful. This individual is in charge of:

1. Documenting roles and task division (determined by the team or team leader).
2. Posting the schedule for the roles that rotate.
3. Reminding team members as needed.

It may also be useful for this person to send an e-mail reminder telling the team who the meeting leader, observer, notetaker, and so on, will be for that week; this is particularly useful if the team has a "team member of the week" (an optional role; see p. 42 for a description), who will need to prepare in advance.

Client Coverage/Team Attendance Manager

The person in this role manages team member absences from team or clinical work. Some or all of these tasks may be important, depending upon the team; teams may also prefer to have existing roles (e.g., team leader, meeting leader) handle these tasks, instead of assigning a separate person to this role. These tasks include:

1. Creating and monitoring a system for tracking team member attendance and absences.

2. Maintaining a policy for client coverage and communicating about such coverage when team members are absent.

3. Monitoring whether team members make their repair to team after an absence, and reminding them to do so when they forget.

Attendance in Team

The team will need a way to monitor attendance in team, in order to detect chronic absences or other attendance problems. This could be completed by the team attendance manager, and/or the notetaker can document team member attendance in the team notes. This could also be tracked by the team leader or another member of the team. In smaller teams, a formal system may not be necessary.

Back-Up Coverage

Many teams need a system for providing back-up coverage within the team. This will vary widely across teams: some teams will not need to address coverage at all (e.g., a residential setting), and some teams may provide full coverage for each other any time a member of the team goes out of town or is otherwise unavailable (e.g., providers in private practice, providers within the same agency). For teams for which this is relevant, a system to request and communicate about back-up coverage can be very useful. The individual in this role can help the team follow the policy for arranging back-up coverage, whatever that policy may be.

In our (JS) team, providers are responsible for finding coverage for their own clients, and must have coverage arranged before leaving town. They request back-up by briefly asking in team or making a request of the team via e-mail. Teammates are quick to volunteer to cover for each other, knowing others will readily cover for them in return. On the rare occasion all team members will be out of town (e.g., for a conference or a holiday), it is recommended that the absent providers maintain phone availability for clients, and find a local licensed DBT provider to provide in-town emergency coverage.

The type of coverage must also be identified. If a teammate is leaving town but is reachable by phone and willing to stay in contact with clients, both of our teams require one person to provide "in-town" coverage, in the event a client needs someone in town for any reason (e.g., a therapy session or other in-person contact is needed). This is very rare but important when needed. If a teammate is leaving town and not accepting client contact while away, the provider will need to request that one or more team members fully cover in their absence, including phone coaching and sessions as needed.

The team must have a way of knowing who is covering for the absent team member. For example, in JS's team, we enter the coverage arrangement in the back-up team member's electronic, secure calendar, so the back-up provider can see clearly when they are on call for another team member's clients. This information is also provided to administrative staff; in the event a client calls the clinic and does not know who the back-up is, the staff can direct the client to the appropriate person. And finally, if the departing provider is not available by phone to clients, they must leave sufficient information for the person providing back-up to cover effectively. In our team, the provider leaves a document, which may be stored on an agency server, a hard copy stored in a secure location, or encrypted and password-protected on another electronic device (e.g., phone) with sufficient client information (name, address, phone number, suicide risk, skills that are most effective for phone or in-session coaching, medications if relevant, other providers if relevant) so that the person providing back-up can coach and communicate with emergency responders effectively. This may also be accomplished through access to a shared electronic medical record, when available.

Whatever the method chosen, if the team is providing back-up coverage, they will need an established system for requesting coverage, assigning coverage for both "in-town" and full coverage, and confidentially communicating client information to the back-up provider. For many teams, the team leader develops this policy, and the individual monitoring absences supports this system; however, this function could be filled by anyone on the team, or even an administrative person. How this process is completed is quite flexible, as long as teams have a system for arranging and communicating about coverage. And once again, each team can decide what components of this arrangement will be useful for them, if any.

Repairing for Team Absence

The other component of this role is that of ensuring repair after a team member misses team. The principle here is to convey the importance of team attendance, and to treat attendance as important as attending therapy sessions. This does not mean team members must be at every single team; vacations are important! But team members do not schedule clients, doctor appointments, phone calls, or other meetings during team time whenever it can be avoided. This is first addressed when orienting and obtaining commitment to join the team, but this culture will need to be maintained on a regular basis. We recommend offering a repair to the team when a teammate is absent, to acknowledge to the team that the absence had an impact on the team. The repair may come in the form of a heartfelt apology, food (spending time baking something, buying treats on the trip, or otherwise showing team the absent teammate was thinking of them), or offering new knowledge acquired while away at a workshop or conference. If the team wishes, the team leader or notetaker could also fulfill the role of noticing absences and reminding each other of the need for repair if someone forgets.

Examples of Additional Roles

Many teams we have worked with have set up additional roles to meet specific functions useful to their particular teams. These are optional, but may be useful to certain teams. Other teams may not require these tasks at all. By including these examples of optional roles, we hope to demonstrate the flexibility and creativity teams can use in setting up their structure.

Room Set-Up

This person will take responsibility for the set-up of the team room, including:

1. Making sure all the necessary forms are copied and in the room (e.g., a blank agenda, meeting leader agreement reminders, observer reminders, blank notes form).
2. Making sure all other materials are present (mindfulness bell,

writing implements, a means to display the previous meeting notes [e.g., a computer and projector]).

3. Turning the computer on.

4. Shredding the agenda and/or other documents at the end of meeting, if necessary.

"Team Member of the Week"

This is a rotating position where one member of the team presents a particular problem (a particular skills deficit or struggle the clinician is experiencing, or a conceptualization of a client who is less acute and does not get mentioned in team frequently) in more detail. This refers to any team member, regardless of their role with the clients. Therefore, every team member will take a turn at "team member of the week" if the team chooses to add this to their agenda. The "team member of the week" typically takes 15 minutes of team time to speak more in depth about a particular difficulty with providing effective care. This allows for team members to obtain consultation on situations that are less likely to be discussed in team, such as agenda items that are lower in urgency and risk and therefore do not get discussed frequently. This also helps the team to become more aware of the provider's case formulation, conceptualization of problems, skills, and responses, and then identify areas for future learning or practice. This role can rotate along with meeting leader, observer, and notetaker if those roles are also rotating weekly, or in a smaller team could occur just once per month. The "team member of the week" still places themselves on the agenda; they may present:

- A video or audio of a particular client–provider interaction.
- A role play of a situation or skill that has proven difficult (the team member may play the role of themselves and/or the client); this may be a problem occurring with a particular client or across clients.
- A case formulation in order to get feedback and shaping (see Rizvi & Sayrs, in press; Koerner, 2012; and Koerner & Linehan, 1997, for case formulation formats).
- A team member may also use the extended time to address a high-risk, time- sensitive issue.

For example, a team member who repeatedly struggles when clients disagree with suggestions could demonstrate the problem via role play, then the team can offer solutions and get the team member to rehearse new behaviors.

Conclusion

In our experience, certain functions are needed for teams to work well. To reiterate, these include managing how time is spent in team, alerting team members to behaviors that deviate from the DBT manual and the team agreements, documenting decisions and suggestions made in team, assigning and rotating roles within the team, providing structure for team member absences, along with any other systems tailored specifically to teams' unique needs. Teams can be flexible in whether and how these are developed and maintained. We have found that the implementation of the above roles is most effective in maintaining the operation of a highly functional DBT team.

IDEAS FOR PRACTICE

- Have a team discussion about which roles might be helpful for your team.
- For one entire team meeting, read through the observer items together as a team after each provider's turn. Briefly discuss which of the items were relevant during the team discussion.
- In each meeting have the team focus only on one observer task. Remain vigilant for that particular behavior throughout the team meeting. For example, for an entire meeting focus carefully on a nonjudgmental stance.
- Rehearse reminding the team to follow the agreements. Each member practices bringing something to the attention of another team member. When practicing, it is not necessary to highlight an actual problem to start; it might help to just practice saying the words to each other. For example, each team member says, "I think you might be judgmental there." Go around the team, with each member repeating the statement.
- Assign one person to be in charge of providing reinforcement for behaviors that maintain the culture of the team. For example, one individual can say, "I'm really glad you brought that up," when one member challenges another member.

The DBT Team Leader

D BT teams need a team leader, a role separate from that of meeting leader (discussed in Chapter 2). The team leader takes the bird's-eye-view of the team and the program as a whole, across time and various goals and problems. This person continuously moves the team toward its visions and values, while maintaining and enhancing the components that are working well. Additionally, the team leader prevents and addresses obstacles to effective team functioning; without such a role, interpersonal, structural, and/or administrative problems may develop.

Sharing leadership duties may not be a problem in a very small team (e.g., two or three people), if there is frequent communication and clear delegation of the responsibilities for making a team work well. For example, the tasks of team leadership could be evenly divided among its members in a small team. As the team and program grow, however, the need for a single person coordinating and tracking these tasks will likely emerge.

What Does "Leadership" Mean?

The six domains of leadership model (Sitkin, Lind, & Siang, 2006; Sitkin & Lind, 2007) provides a useful structure for leadership in the DBT team. This model draws a distinction between a leader and a manager in the workplace. A manager, by their definition, is one who implements authority and control over employees, using the employees' own individual self-interest to utilize incentives or other means to get them to behave in certain ways. While this may be an important role in any workplace, this is *not* what is meant by the DBT team's team leader. In contrast, a leader by their definition is one who gets individuals focused more on communal interests and a common vision through the connection to the group. The focus on the team and shared goals is thought to inspire and persuade individuals to choose to behave in certain ways, rather than relying on measures of control. This form of leading is essential in a DBT team; if management is necessary, it is better conducted through a different means such as supervision or an employer–employee relationship. In order to set up the trust, vulnerability, and respect needed in a DBT team, leadership, not management, is necessary within the DBT team.

This isn't to say that team leaders don't use contingencies and other methods to influence behavior, nor does it mean that leaders are not also fulfilling the roles of managers, bosses, employers, and supervisors. However, in a DBT team, if a leader acts as only a manager by controlling team members, it can result in members hiding mistakes, not communicating, and ultimately undermining the goals and agreements of the team.

The six domains of leadership model suggests a set of skills that is necessary to lead, which is also useful for leading a DBT team. In brief, these skills include:

1. Personal leadership: leading with authenticity and expertise, from one's own personality and values.

2. Relational leadership: conveying that one cares about those they lead, sees them as real people, with respect and understanding, building reciprocal trust between the leader and those they lead.

3. Contextual leadership: building a coherent team identity with a sense of community.

4. Inspirational leadership: encouraging enthusiasm and optimism, while maintaining high expectations.

5. Supportive leadership: providing the resources and belief in every individual's ability to respond effectively to problems, ensure the members have the training, resources, and encouragement needed, while working to eliminate blame or take the blame themselves if a solution is not effective.

6. Responsible leadership: leading with ethics, representing the team values in their public role, and balancing individual and team needs successfully.

Beyond the leadership skills listed above, additional characteristics are uniquely useful for a DBT leader. First, leading a DBT team requires a certain vulnerability, willingness, and "we're in the trenches together" approach. Such equality is a characteristic principle of DBT and the DBT team that may not be present in other settings. This vulnerability is discussed later in this chapter.

Second, this individual must enter into the position willingly, with enthusiasm and dedication. The most experienced, best-trained DBT clinician will not make an effective team leader in the absence of a true dedication to leading the DBT team. This role requires persistence and willingness to guide the team in solving difficult problems. In some teams, the person with the most expertise may not be the best team leader.

Finally, and perhaps most importantly, this person must also engage DBT principles and strategies sufficiently to lead. Depending on the setting, multiple facets might be required to fulfill this role. While not a complete list, the examples below illustrate how DBT expertise can benefit the leader and team.

- Overall knowledge of and experience with DBT treatment can be extremely helpful in order to build respect from team members and the larger agency, if relevant.

- The ability to take a dialectical stance, balancing acceptance and change in the team and for the program as a whole, will help the leader manage the team's, team members', and clients' needs.

- Mindfulness skills help the leader to bring full attention to the team, see the team as a whole with clarity and wisdom and without judgment, respond to difficult situations, and effectively attend to the team and clients. These skills also help the team leader remain mindful of each individual's learning process, skillfully support members, and respond to their mistakes and challenges effectively.

- Distress Tolerance and Emotion Regulation skills facilitate effective leader response to team problems, such as complaints made about leadership, disappointment in a course of events, or grieving a loss. Leaders must be able to tolerate their own distress while simultaneously leading the team and each team member in dealing with their own emotions and distress.

- Interpersonal Effectiveness skills can help the leader shape team-mates' behavior without significantly damaging their motivation. The leader will also find these skills are essential to obtain support from agency administration, if relevant. The team leader may also need to manage strong opinions in team, particularly if there are multiple experts in team.

As mentioned above, the role of team leader is separate from that of meeting leader, who monitors meeting time and the agenda; the team leader watches over the program as a whole. This role cannot switch week to week or month to month; this role requires continuity and a certain level of dedication to the team that goes above and beyond what is required of other team members. This individual may have an administrative role, may be other team members' boss and/or clinical supervisor, may have financial or other kinds of power over others, and/or may be the most experienced person on team. Or it may not be those individuals; it may simply be the person who is most enthusiastic about DBT and willing to take on the task.

Tasks of the DBT Team Leader

The leader's central job is to monitor and enhance clients' well-being, team members' well-being, and the effectiveness of the overall program. The scope of leadership and the specific job description may look very different based on the goals of the team. Once again, the team will do best if the leader's tasks are mindfully and strategically chosen, rather than copying another team's structure or following certain "rules." Ideally, the leader functions to set and maintain a structure that both enhances DBT and removes obstacles from team members, so they can do their clinical jobs as efficiently and skillfully as possible. The leader can coordinate the system such that the program remains viable and each team member is best able to provide effective treatment. By having eyes on problems before they develop, the leader provides an environment that facilitates DBT. While the leader does not need to single-handedly solve any of these problems, it is essential to be monitoring and wrestling with these problems before they grow beyond repair, focusing on what will be helpful to the team, program, and agency. It is hoped that the team leader's role provides a sense of freedom and flexibility for team members, rather than a sense of control and constriction.

Tasks will also vary by the type of setting in which the team functions. If the team is made up of several providers in private practice, the team leader may have fewer responsibilities; if the team leader is also the administrative leader for the program, it may include many more. If nestled in an agency or larger company, some of the team leader's tasks may be established by the administration and may not be under the direct control of the leader or team. Across a variety of settings, the tasks of the leader may include:

1. Addressing team cohesion, enthusiasm, health, and problems.
2. Addressing team members' well-being.
3. Addressing team logistics.
4. Addressing program logistics, program well-being, and client complaints.
5. Managing public relations.
6. Interacting with administration and others in the environment/ system.
7. Recruiting new team members.
8. Removing someone from the team.
9. Monitoring and managing contingencies.

These areas are often interconnected, but for the sake of clarity we will discuss each in turn.

Addressing Team Cohesion, Enthusiasm, Health, and Problems

The team leader will be central to maintaining a caring, supportive atmosphere in team, which can generate resiliency for times when problems arise. Motivating a team might consist of sharing reports of successful clients or reminding the team of the beneficial impact the treatment is having. It might be simply demonstrating love for the clients and the work, or struggling openly with certain clinical situations, just as other team members do. It could be praise, support, and gifts of chocolate. It could be a phone call to check in with a certain team member when times are hard. The leader can introduce an element of fun to team as well. Other team members may respond well to reminders of how noble the work is, how effective the treatment is, and how important the providers' efforts are. Focusing on the rationale of the agreements is useful as well; team members may not enjoy being instructed to be nonjudgmental repeatedly but being reminded of why it is helpful to drop the judgments may be extremely motivating. Team members will vary widely in what works for them. A team discussion about what inspires, what motivates, and what keeps DBT providers going is helpful. And once again, while the leader's inspiration and motivation are essential, the entire team will benefit from attempting to inspire each other, rather than waiting for the leader to take this task on alone. This topic will be addressed again later in this chapter, regarding *how* a team leader can effectively behave in team.

Relatedly, leaders will be most helpful to their teams if they can manage their own distress well. Leaders who are burned out; judgmental of the team, clients, or treatment; or otherwise modeling a lack of enthusiasm can create a contagion effect. This is not to say that leaders must be incredibly charismatic, nor solely responsible for their team's happiness. But leaders with dedication and evident enthusiasm will likely grow that sentiment in their teams, whereas leaders who are frustrated and burned out may generate more of that emotion in team.

Solving current problems and anticipating future problems are both an important part of the team leader's role. Having a team leader take the pulse of the team from time to time, as discussed in Chapter 6, may allow for earlier intervention. The leader is also the one who, upon discovering a team problem, determines whether it is worth taking the time to address and solve the problem, remembering that not all problems must be solved. The team leader is in a position to see patterns developing over time (as opposed to the observer, which as a rotating role may not have the same perspective) and can make a master plan for if and how to tackle the problem. When a difficult problem does not resolve successfully, it is the team leader who manages the challenge and continues to guide the team in finding a solution. All of this is done with input from the team as needed.

For example, over time teams may lose the synthesis of acceptance and change, and more specifically, motivation and fidelity. In other words, teams may focus so much on fidelity that team interactions lose warmth and support, or at the other extreme, teams may validate in the absence of pushing each other for change. Ideally, the entire team will monitor this potential problem, but the leader can help the team by identifying such problems early and guiding the team toward intervention. When the team leans toward more validation and support, the leader can highlight the need for change strategies; when too much focus is on change and a team member is becoming demoralized, the leader can highlight the need for increased support and validation. In either case, the leader can suggest discussions, structural changes, exercises, or other interventions to help address the imbalance. The observer and the other members will also watch for this; maintaining the dialectic is the whole team's job.

Interpersonal problems may develop as well; for example, one teammate might repeatedly take more time than allotted, and when the meeting leader asks them to wrap up to allow the next person to take a turn, the teammate becomes visibly distressed. At first, team members might be flexible and supportive, but over time perhaps become more frustrated, and display subtle signs of judgment, such as eye rolling or looking at each other when they become distressed. While the observer may not catch the developing pattern over time due to the rotating role, the leader (and other members) may notice the gradual change. The leader may not feel the need to intervene at first, but once the pattern is evident, they can try a variety of strategies that might include highlighting the problem, asking the team if there is an elephant in the room and/or to use a nonjudgmental stance, and asking the individual to request more time and/or tolerate the time limit. Again, these interventions are chosen based on what seems most effective for the team; the leader and others can use much flexibility in how to respond.

The leader may also provide assistance when a team becomes polarized or stuck on a particular issue. For example, two members may disagree regarding the course of treatment for a client and be unable to find a synthesis. The team has several mechanisms for such problems, including speaking directly with each other and utilizing the role of the observer, but at times the leader will need to intervene to move the situation forward. Because the leader is monitoring team health, and may be approached by team members when there are difficulties, the leader may become aware of problems before others on the team. The leader and individual member(s) will then need to decide whether the topic should be discussed in team or outside of team.

And most importantly, likely no one will be satisfied with a team that solves problems well but doesn't have *fun* together. The leader can support a sense of community, enjoyment, even silliness, in team. The leader can also schedule social time with team, such as dinners, retreats, happy hour, and so on. The team will fare the best if everyone contributes to this culture, but the leader may have the ability to provide a budget, organization, and dedication to making sure the team goes beyond managing problems to being a team everyone looks forward to seeing. Asking team members what would make and keep them happy, and responding within reason, can go a long way toward keeping individuals, and therefore the team as a whole, satisfied and productive.

Addressing Team Members' Well-Being

Relatedly, team leaders will address *individual* team members' well-being and problems in some settings. In team, the leader may notice a single member who is creating challenges for the team; this might include a chronically judgmental teammate, or one who repeatedly describes clients in nonbehavioral terms. There may also be problems with one member feeling judged, or not liking team, or not liking particular people in team. Oftentimes this is very straightforward (although not always easy!); the leader (and others in the team) can highlight the pattern, assess, and work toward solutions.

It is not always feasible or wise to bring up every individual problem in the team; having a leader with whom to speak privately, brainstorm ideas, share dissatisfaction or burnout, and get help in making adjustments to the job description, caseload, or other arrangements may be highly useful. Not everyone will need to come to the leader in this regard, but knowing the team leader is available to talk to when one is feeling dissatisfied can be important in itself. This may be especially true when the team leader is also the supervisor or boss of team members. The team leader will need to use caution with this information. Team members may provide the team leader with highly sensitive, confidential information, such as that they are thinking of leaving the program or have made a serious mistake with a client. If the leader's response is aversive, or if the leader discloses the information to the team without the member's collaboration, they may not disclose again, so remaining mindful of the impact of one's response is important.

A team member may come to the leader in private to discuss

difficulty with the behavior of a particular team member (either problems in adhering to DBT or simply disliking a person). In these situations, the DBT dialectic of consultation to the patient and environmental intervention is very relevant. In DBT, providers act as consultants to the client, which means providing coaching and suggestions but not intervening for the client, as often as possible. On the other hand, there are situations where it is worth the lost opportunity for learning to move in and intervene for the client in the client's environment. This dialectic is discussed at length within DBT (Linehan, 1993). This principle is helpful to DBT team leaders as well: in most situations, if a team member approaches the team leader for help with another member, the leader can be a consultant, providing suggestions and ideas but not solving the problem for the team member. There will be situations, however, when power, status, personality, failure of previous solutions, or other factors may make it worth an environmental intervention from the leader. This decision requires a great deal of mindfulness about the consequences of the intervention for all involved.

For example, a new member of a team I (JS) worked with was very hurt by an experienced teammate. She approached the team leader outside of team because she was afraid of challenging this experienced person in front of everyone. With my help, she did pros and cons of speaking to her directly, she role-played what she would say, then finally she spoke to this individual outside of team. (She chose to do so outside of team, but others might choose to do so in team; as long as the situation is being addressed, there are no hard rules about where this problem is discussed.) In another situation, a teammate became quite angry and made repeated comments to particular members of the team that were experienced as very hurtful. There were multiple attempts to address this problem directly in team, which were met with more of the same comments. In this case, the leader intervened, met with the individual alone, and asked what was going on. It was not until the one-on-one conversation that the problem was effectively addressed.

The leader can also remove obstacles for team members when possible. The dialectic of consultation to the team member and environmental intervention is still very relevant, but team members will be more motivated, more energized, and more excited about clinical care if the leader can smooth the way. For example, in a team where a member is experiencing a particularly stressful clinical situation, the leader might offer to give live coaching while the provider is in contact with the client, provide coverage for other clients, bring the teammate lunch, or arrange other help within the team. (And once again, the entire team can help!) Being able to identify problems early, facilitate solution generation and implementation, and simply make life as a clinician easier for individual team members can go a long way toward maintaining teammates' well-being.

Addressing Team Logistics

The team leader may also be placed in charge of team logistics. This job may include setting the start time and length of the team meeting, which client is assigned to whom, and the team structure. The leader may choose a particular agenda format, set the team schedule, and ensure other roles are assigned and fulfilled. Sometimes the team will need items purchased, such as props or books for the treatment or the team; the leader may be in charge of obtaining those items. If there is a team budget of any kind, the leader may be in charge of monitoring the funds and discussing with the team how that money might be spent (training, social time, etc.). In a team where it is difficult to arrange clinical coverage for vacations, the leader might improve the coverage system or provide reinforcers for those offering to cover, to facilitate regular vacations for team members.

Addressing Program Logistics

This set of tasks may vary widely depending on the type of setting. Leaders may set policies regarding what types of clients are seen or referred out, pursue team goals such as adding a client population to the program's areas of competence, hire, fire, set program policies regarding fees and financial guidelines, manage legal issues/consultation, and create clinic rules. In an independent clinic, the team leader will likely be in charge of all of these jobs, plus possibly marketing, business taxes, payroll, and so on; in a hospital setting, the team leader will have a narrower scope, but may spend significant time communicating with those higher in the administration to pave the way for program development and changes. In a group of private practitioners, the leader may have none of these tasks. In any setting, the leader can look for ways to monitor the effectiveness of the program through client satisfaction, client outcome, or other means to confirm the program is indeed providing effective services. Handling client complaints is another task that may fall to the leader, as well as helping a client switch individual therapists or skills groups when it is deemed effective to do so.

Interacting with Administration and Others in the Environment/System

Team leaders may also be the liaison between the DBT team and the administration and/or others in the program's larger system. Such a position may require the team leader to deal with requests from the administration to change certain elements of the DBT program. The team leader may not have the freedom to make decisions for the team but must obtain approval from those making policy or budget decisions elsewhere in the agency. For example, many team leaders may need to convince administration that DBT skills groups require a leader and a coleader, team members must join voluntarily, clients must enter DBT voluntarily, not every client needs DBT, phone coaching is a necessary part of treatment, or skills groups must have a size limit. Budget restrictions or other policies may interfere with the DBT team adhering to the manual in these and other ways. The team leader, therefore, must implement skills and knowledge when communicating with administration, whether it is a hospital budget committee, an owner of a clinic, a board of directors, or any other setting where the person designing the program is not trained in DBT, to get the program to adherence. The team leader helps to make sure the system provides the team what it needs to function effectively, balancing protecting the culture of the team with responding to the administration's requirements, requesting changes from administration as necessary. Many skills may be needed to manage this (at times very challenging) task, including:

1. *Interpersonal Effectiveness skills.* Knowing how to ask the administration for what the team needs skillfully, adjust intensity of communication effectively, preserve the relationship while getting what one wants, and a variety of other skills from the Interpersonal Effectiveness module will be very helpful.

2. *Understanding what the reinforcers are for the administrators.* In other words, what motivates the individuals who are creating policies and running budgets in this setting? The team leader will need to spend

time with the administrators, develop relationships, understand the pressures placed on them, and see the DBT team from the administrators' perspective. The leader can also make sure the DBT team can provide reinforcers, rather than added strain and difficulty for the administrators, as often as possible. As with any relationship, one must assess rather than assume what the reinforcers might be. Reinforcers may include:

a. *Providing excellent care.* Many mental health center owners and administrators are highly motivated by providing excellent care, particularly to those who are unable to receive effective care elsewhere, which often includes DBT clients. Reminding administrators of the data supporting the efficacy of DBT can be very powerful in getting them to support the treatment in its entirety, as it is described in the manual and as it has been studied in prestigious research trials. Also, informing administrators of the achievements of the team can be very useful; this information might include feedback from clients or other providers, teaching, publications, invited presentations, and the development of outreach or other innovative programs.

b. *Documenting outcomes of excellent care.* Relatedly, providing administrators with data about the DBT program's own clients, including number of visits to the ER, suicide attempts, self-harm incidents, and so on, can be very motivating to those making policy and budget decisions for the DBT program. Comparisons to clients' rates of problem behaviors prior to attending DBT, such as from their intake interview or previous records, can demonstrate the impact the DBT program is having on these clients, many of whom may consume resources at a higher rate than non-DBT clients.

c. *Reducing liability.* If administrators attempt to cut parts of the DBT program in order to save money (e.g., decrease team time or skills group time, eliminate one group leader), it can be very helpful to remind administrators that DBT is an evidence-based treatment, and once elements are removed from the treatment, it is no longer based on the evidence. If there were to be a lawsuit against the agency or particular team member, for example, providing the treatment as the manual states and as the evidence suggests may provide some protection. If administrators understand the agency's liability could be increased by veering from the DBT manual, they may be more likely to support the DBT team's needs in providing the treatment according to the manual. Making these arguments to the administrators will require that the team leader knows the DBT manuals and the data supporting DBT very well.

   d. *Saving money.* Administrators will often be highly influenced by saving money. Depending upon the setting, administrators may be very interested to learn that providing DBT can actually save the agency money, compared to treating certain clients with an alternative, nonmanualized treatment. Administrators are under pressure themselves to fit programs in certain budgets. Presenting administrators with DBT's cost-effectiveness data (e.g., Krawitz & Miga, 2019; Haga, Aas, Groholt, Tormoen, & Mehlum, 2018; Pasieczny & Connor, 2011; Linehan & Heard, 1999) related to providing adherent DBT can be very powerful in increasing their willingness to allot resources to the DBT team.

   e. *Making money.* Not only are administrators trying to save money, they are often highly motivated to make money. Demonstrating how the DBT team contributes to the financial health of the overall organization will be essential. For example, a DBT program that keeps providers' caseloads full, maintains the program at a size that supports the agency budget, provides referrals to other providers in the agency, and sets fees so the program helps the bottom line will all be important in getting administrators to support and protect the DBT program.

   f. *Reducing turnover in staff.* Staff turnover is costly to any business; when staff become burned out or enticed by other job offers, it will have a detrimental impact financially. Administrators will be motivated by interventions that keep staff happy and productive. If the team leader can make a strong case for the ways DBT, and the DBT team in particular, stave off burnout and increase the well-being and performance of its members, and therefore reduce the need to replace providers, this may enhance administrators' support for policies that are beneficial to the team. This may also be true for reasonable salaries, adequate time off, time for team, paid training, or being paid for coaching clients outside of session.

   g. *Enhancing the agency's reputation in the community.* If the DBT team leader can demonstrate to the administration that the DBT team is providing leading-edge treatment that is following the emerging science, and that doing so is enhancing the reputation of the agency at large in the community, administration may be more prone to support the DBT program. The DBT team leader can play a key part in this role by educating other providers in the area through presentations, consultations, and informal interactions with other providers. As the agency comes to be known as the place to go for the best care, the entire agency will benefit from the DBT program's excellent services, which will in turn garner more administrative support.

3. *Remaining nonjudgmental and dialectical, and looking for what is being left out.* When administrator decisions seem nonsensical, this means the team leader is missing information. Administrators may have different goals and different values than the clinicians in the DBT team, but there *are* reasons for the decisions made at a higher administrative level, even if the team leader disagrees with those reasons. When team leaders become judgmental and polarized, they will miss valuable information, and may spread discontent throughout the team. Nonjudgmentally questioning what information is being left out and asking how such an administrative decision makes sense without attachment to what is "right" can help the leader gain a much better understanding of the decisions made about policies and budgets. This can open up new alternatives for solving team problems within the given parameters, and to pave the way for important changes to be made.

Managing Public Relations

Any program will need client flow. In some teams, the leader is the point-person for communicating with local professionals, keeping the program name well known, marketing, and bringing in clients. This can be a sizable and stressful job, depending on the size of the program; in large cities within a well-known hospital, this may be less of a task, but for independent programs, the leader may monitor client flow, connect with other professionals, and request that teammates network as well. Once again, delegating and getting team help with this task may be very useful, but having a leader to monitor and organize the task will likely be necessary in certain settings. In private practice settings, the team can discuss what types of networking may be useful to keep caseloads full. With well-established programs/providers, this task may not be necessary at all.

Recruiting New Team Members

In some settings, the team leader will be responsible for recruiting new team members. This job might include placing ads, arranging interviews, screening candidates, and arranging for the commitment session discussed in Chapter 8. The leader will not select a new team member without input; the agency may have some investment in this decision, and the team members will ideally be closely involved in this process.

Removing Someone from the Team

In rare situations, one individual in the team may become unwilling or unable to follow the team agreements. Much as in DBT, the team leader can try a number of strategies to turn the situation around, along with all members of the team; only after these strategies have been tried will the possibility of asking an individual to leave the team arise. Assessing and attempting to solve the problem may prevent more serious measures from being taken. There are several strategies for a situation where one team member is not following the agreements:

1. Bring up the problem in team, and/or the leader may bring up the problem one-on-one with the individual.
2. Identify the specific problem that is interfering, with a very concrete definition of the problem behavior and the team agreement that needs work.
3. Assess; attempt to identify controlling variables.
4. Identify solutions.
5. Obtain commitment.
6. Troubleshoot.
7. If these strategies are unsuccessful, teams may also ask a consultant to join the team for a period of time, in order to facilitate an intervention.

When these strategies do not work, it will likely be the leader's job to make a decision about when to ask this person to leave the team. There will be times when the health of the team depends on the leader making this decision, such as when one individual has become sufficiently judgmental of the team, treatment, or clients that it is harming others.

Moving through this process in a kind, compassionate, supportive manner will help to buffer all involved from the emotional consequences this type of process might entail.

The leader may be tempted to ignore the problem or to avoid conflict; however, this can be extremely damaging to team morale in certain situations. Many of these problems can be prevented if the leader makes careful choices about who will join the team, implements effective commitment strategies, and establishes a healthy team culture, but these strategies do not completely protect a team from one individual creating significant damage. On the other hand, some problems can be safely ignored. It will be up to the leader's judgment to determine whether the behavior is interfering with team functioning and not solvable in other ways.

For example, we consulted to a team where one member was burned out, angry, and very distressed. She became very judgmental and detached in team, dismissing feedback from teammates. She paid less attention, made judgmental comments and facial expressions (e.g., eye rolls), and did not ask for or accept consultation from teammates. The observer and other team members highlighted her behavior, noting that her judgmental attitude and other behaviors were interfering with team functioning. The team attempted to assess the problem, but she was unwilling to discuss the problem in team. The team leader determined that all this behavior interfered sufficiently with team functioning and that additional intervention was needed, and therefore met with her individually. The leader attempted to pinpoint the obstacles to engaging in team, but she again was not willing to discuss or try to solve the problem. After much deliberation, the leader then told her that she needed to show some willingness to change particular behaviors, or the leader would consider asking her to leave the team. She gave it serious thought and then chose to leave the team herself. Because of the leader's skill, she was able to leave amicably and with enough notice that clients had time to switch to new individual therapists in a thoughtful manner.

This process can also involve a temporary break, similar to the idea of a therapeutic vacation in DBT. In DBT treatment, when clients are unwilling to work toward clinical goals, the individual therapist along with the team may, as a last resort before ending treatment altogether, suspend treatment temporarily (as opposed to permanently) until the client is willing and engaged. Similarly, in team, the leader may choose to temporarily suspend membership until problems are addressed.

These decisions must be made very thoughtfully, as losing a teammate is distressing to the team and to clients, but the DBT team's format and goals are not for everyone, and those who are unwilling or
unable to work within the team agreements may no longer be given
the option of remaining on the team. And while the entire team is
responsible for highlighting problems, it may ultimately come down to
the team leader to make this difficult decision. Depending on the setting, those clients may either remain with that provider but no longer
be treated by the team (e.g., when that person is in independent private
practice), or be transferred to other DBT individual therapists in the
team (in an agency or group setting where all DBT clients are seen on
this team, and the teammate must leave clients behind when departing
from the team).

Joining a DBT team is voluntary and requires a willingness to
embrace the assumptions, agreements, and DBT itself. At times an
agency may require a staff person to join the team when the staff member
is not entering voluntarily. The leader will need to be very active in this
situation. Meeting with the staff person and determining the level of willingness to follow the agreements will be an important first step. Informing the administration of the cons to placing a nonvoluntary member on
the team will also be essential (e.g., it can significantly impact the quality
of client care, team satisfaction, and staff retention). See Chapter 8 for a
discussion of voluntary membership.

Even with a fully voluntary team, commitment may wane for some
individuals; the leader will need to protect clients and the team by
actively intervening. Asking someone to leave should be a last resort but
is a necessary course of action in certain circumstances. Exiting from the
team is not done as a punishment, but as a natural outcome of decreased
dedication to or interest in the team mission.

Monitoring and Managing Contingencies

Due to their position of relative power and visibility, team leaders will
be providing contingencies throughout team, whether they are aware of
this or not. It is therefore very important to be mindful of these contingencies, and to manage them skillfully. Leaders have particularly strong
reinforcers at their disposal (e.g., praise from leaders may be stronger than
praise from another member of team), and disapproval from leaders may
function as a more potent punisher. Leaders can inadvertently shape

ineffective behaviors in team members if they do not remain aware of these contingencies.

For example, I (JS) was consulting to a team that was struggling with developing a culture of openness and vulnerability. As part of developing this new culture, one team member shared that she had made a mistake with a client and could use help to avoid the problem in the future. The leader immediately became (quite understandably) frightened that one of her team members had said something problematic to a client, and started to tell this provider why that should never happen and that she must never do it again. While this response did make the leader feel somewhat reassured, it actually punished any admission on this provider's part, as well as other teammates who learned from this interaction that it was not safe to admit mistakes. As we discussed this process together, the leader shared that she had a moment of emotion and failed to be mindful of the aversive consequence she delivered and the message sent to all the team members. We discussed how she might instead reinforce the admission with a calm demeanor, express gratitude for the provider's willingness to be open with the team, and provide helpful suggestions, all of which could increase the likelihood that all team members would share and request help when they made mistakes.

It can be very difficult to reinforce certain behaviors in team. For example, when a team member says, "I think you might have drifted from the treatment model," the team leader and all members will need to provide reinforcement, such as, "Thank you for saying so. Tell me more," or "I'm so glad you pointed that out!" If the leader wants team members not only to support teammates, but also to challenge them, then any time an individual highlights a concern, it will be beneficial to provide reinforcement and to remind other members to do so as well. When a member is highlighting the dialectic by pointing out the validity in a different perspective, the team leader can notice and appreciate the dialectical stance, rather than immediately disagreeing. The leader, in particular, will need the mindfulness skills to identify behaviors that are in line with the team agreements, and highlight this for the whole team as effective behavior. The team leader can suggest that the entire team remain mindful of this need, as well.

There can be a very subtle process in team whereby a leader can reinforce "apparent competence," (Linehan, 1993), or the apparent skillfulness of team members. Apparent competence is a term used in DBT when one's appearance or words do not match one's experience. In other words, one looks "fine" or skillful when one is actually struggling and not "fine." It may be more challenging to identify difficulties in front of the team leader, due to this phenomenon; leaders (as well as other teammates) can be so comforted by someone looking like they know what they're doing, they can fail to realize that an individual, intentionally or not, is presenting as more skillful than they feel, or presenting as more competent than is warranted. As other members see very competent-looking individuals receive a lot of reinforcement from the leader and team, they may feel they need to present as very competent as well, meaning fewer mistakes, emotions, and other vulnerabilities are displayed in team. This again can present a problem for team functioning. Team leaders' reactions to team problems are essential to monitor in these situations. Responding with distress, correction, and/or invalidation to the member who shows vulnerability, or disproportionately more attention and praise to those who do not show vulnerability, can inadvertently shape a team toward certain responses. The leader and all members can watch for this pattern, and aim to reinforce vulnerability, not just competence.

A word of caution in applying contingencies to team members' behavior: this could once again move the team leader into the role of expert, teacher, or some other one-up position (see dialectical dilemmas on pp. 64–65). The contingencies the leader applies (e.g., reinforcing direct conversation in team; discussing late arrivals to team) will hopefully be applied by other team members as well. This is difficult, because other team members may not want to challenge someone who is late or enforce an agreement. But if the team relies solely on the leader to do this work, and the leader fills this role alone, the team is no longer functioning within the structure of a DBT team. The leader or any other team member may highlight this drift from DBT, and all team members ideally would work together to return to the team structure and agreements.

What Is *Not* the Leader's Job?

While the leader has many responsibilities within the DBT team, *it is not the leader's job to solve everything.* The burden of highlighting and solving problems remains with the entire team, as does the task of getting the team activated and using strategies. The leader's job is to step in, bring the problem to the attention of the team, and plan what type of intervention is needed, when the team fails to do so itself. For most problems, all members of the team must participate to solve the problem in a way that helps the team function effectively. The leader must stay alert, facilitate change within the team, yet not solve everything alone.

Relatedly, it is not the leader's job to control other members. We have seen many leaders who, out of anxiety for the clients or themselves, feel a strong urge to control exactly how teammates handle clinical situations and dominate the team. Again, this affects the team culture and can create several problems. Leaders do have an obligation to say something when they believe a clinician has veered from effective care, but moving into a controlling role can significantly change the team dynamic. This is even more difficult to navigate when leaders are also bosses, supervisors, and otherwise responsible and even liable for team members' behavior. We find it is best to leave those roles outside of team. If a leader is supervising someone on their own license, the leader and supervisee should meet regularly outside of team to review clinical care. In the team, the leader may provide suggestions, even strongly assert someone do or not do something, but cannot control team members. The team is a place to provide and receive consultation, and to conduct therapy for the therapist. The primary goal is to help teammates wrestle with feedback and come back to wise mind decisions with the client. Controlling team members will interfere with both the clinicians thinking for themselves and the team functioning well.

It is also not the leader's job to make decisions based on liability. In our experience, fear of being liable for leading a DBT team can lead to unskillful, emotion mind-based decisions. Doing DBT and running a DBT team can offer their own protection, in that the team members are offering state-of-the-science treatment, and clients are receiving the best treatment the evidence can offer. But fear can still arise; allowing fear to unduly influence decisions is not helpful. If a leader or other team members notice a team member missing something important with respect to client care or risk, they would of course say something, and may even meet one-on-one with the team member to emphasize the importance of a particular intervention, but the leader would ideally do so from wise mind not emotion mind. Team leaders must use all the DBT skills to regulate any emotion related to liability or other concerns, remain in wise mind, radically accept that this work inevitably involves some risk, then move the focus back to providing solid DBT and running an effective DBT team.

And finally, all of these recommendations are balanced with the notion that the team leader is absolutely not expected to be perfect. Just as we are all expected to make a lot of mistakes in our clinical work, team leaders are also expected to make a lot of mistakes in leading their DBT teams. It is extremely challenging to lead a group of individuals doing very intense, difficult work, and impossible to make everyone happy all the time. The team leader and team members can practice tolerating mistakes, experiencing interpersonal tension, working toward solving problems, and allowing for imperfection. One does not need to attain all of the recommendations in this chapter; skillful means points the way to prioritizing, working hard on the areas that are most important, and practicing radical acceptance that not all issues will find a resolution, or at least an immediate one. The DBT team will thrive if the team leader can set a course for the most effective team possible, remaining open to feedback, suggestions, and even complaints, while maintaining consistency and shaping the course for the entire team.

Dialectical Dilemmas for Team Leaders

Team leaders will likely experience a number of dialectical tensions, in which they are faced with two opposing forces that appear impossible to navigate. The leader may feel pressured to weigh both sides and choose one pole, leaving the other pole unaddressed. Within a dialectical framework, however, the team leader searches for and finds the validity in both poles, and in doing so comes to a synthesis, or a new standpoint from which to view the problem. The synthesis may lead to new ideas, solutions, and pathways for moving forward. The synthesis is not a compromise, nor a diluted version of each extreme; it involves fully embodying each extreme, allowing them to coexist, then moving forward. And moving forward does not require a resolution; at times the team leader and the team can simply hold both poles and allow the tension between the two to exist without a resolution.

The most frequently referenced dialectic in DBT is that of acceptance and change. As discussed previously, DBT providers do not choose between acceptance and change; nor do they accept at certain times and ask for change at different times. Instead, DBT clinicians deeply understand and accept their clients, exactly as they are, wholly and unconditionally, *and* are fully aware of the necessity of change in every moment.

Both poles are intensely true in DBT. The expression of this tension may look different at different points in the treatment (e.g., the provider may work for change for an entire session, or may alternate rapidly between validating and problem solving, or may validate for an extended period), but the clinician is not choosing between the poles and instead is embodying both in every moment.

The team leader will also be presented with difficult tensions in the leadership position, and just as in DBT treatment, will be most effective if they can embody both poles fully rather than choosing one pole over the other. The team leader's dialectical dilemmas, illustrated in Figure 3.1, are best described as dimensions defined by their opposite poles. The overarching dilemma for DBT team leaders is also that of acceptance versus change within the team. Within this larger dialectic, common tensions include: (1) modeling vulnerability versus modeling expertise; (2) being a team member versus being a team leader; and (3) attending to other needs (e.g., for a specific team member or client; for the agency) versus attending to the team's needs. Not all team leaders will experience all of the dialectical dilemmas presented here. Depending upon the setting and the scope of the team leader's tasks, only some of these tensions may apply to any particular team, and leaders may observe additional tensions emerging.

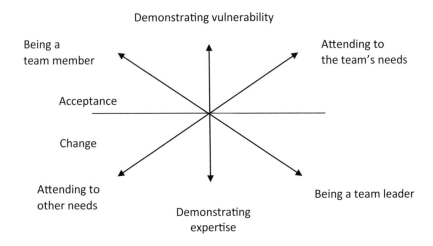

FIGURE 3.1. Dialectical dilemmas for DBT team leaders.

Acceptance of Team Members versus Changing Team Members

DBT teams are, at their core, change-oriented. The team's purpose and function is to strive for the most effective DBT treatment possible, and to remain within a dialectical perspective. Fulfilling these tasks requires team members to constantly challenge each other, question each other's decisions, remind each other of the agreements, and highlight opportunities to improve. This is, by nature, very change-focused. While much of the onus for such change falls on the observer and all members of the team, the leader will play an important role by making adjustments in team culture and structure as needed to fulfill its purpose.

If a team and team leader focus nondialectically on change, however, the team will stray from its dialectical stance. Without a synthesis of acceptance and change, team members can feel invalidated, unsupported, frustrated by the change focus, or even hopeless about their ability to improve; team members may not want to be corrected repeatedly, or for the leader to have the final word in every discussion. Team members may stop sharing, which will be counter to the team agreements. Team members also need to experience an acceptance of their current struggles, the slow pace of change, and the fact that it will not be possible to solve many of their clients' and their own problems overnight. Team members will need validation that their difficulties make sense and are normative, as well as praise for their efforts. The focus on acceptance is essential to provide an environment where teammates are willing to be vulnerable, discuss mistakes, express emotion, and look forward to attending and fully participating in team meetings.

On the other hand, if provided nondialectically, acceptance in isolation can also create problems for a DBT team. Team members can drift away from the manual when there is no mechanism for highlighting and changing such drift. Team members can be reinforced for providing ineffective therapy. The agreements and the manual will cease to have influence over time, if one is in a team that provides acceptance without change.

While the acceptance and change synthesis is not solely the responsibility of the team leader (but that of the whole team), the team leader will have significant influence over the culture of the team. Synthesizing acceptance and change can become a core part of the team's culture if the team leader and other members can implement such a synthesis in every team meeting. Just as a DBT provider does with clients, the team leader can model deeply understanding and accepting a struggle a teammate discusses, while at the same time emphasizing the importance of changing, solving, and moving the team member forward. This may take on different appearances in different discussions; for example, a team member may only need validation at times, or may not need any validation at all and wants only solutions. Emphasizing this dialectic will be essential for the team as a whole to strike an effective, flexible balance.

Demonstrating Vulnerability versus Demonstrating Expertise

At one pole, it is useful for the team leader to exhibit expertise and fidelity whenever possible. The team leader is a model for the team, whether they are aware of that or not. The team will likely find comfort and reassurance in a strong leader who embodies DBT principles and has ideas and answers for difficult consultation questions. Following the agreements, such as arriving on time, will convey the value of doing so to other members and help to establish the cultural norm. The team leader can monitor and maintain all of the agreements as much as possible, so they are maintained within the team culture. Team members will also look to the leader to determine how to follow the DBT manual, how flexible to be, how seriously the commitment to team will be taken, and whether the DBT and team manuals are rigidly held or considered a set of principles that one mindfully follows. A leader who tells others to be on time but arrives late sends the message that being on time is not important; a leader who does not work at being less judgmental communicates that judgments are acceptable in team; a leader who does not emphasize the importance of following the data and remaining mindful of the DBT manual could contribute to an entire team drifting away from DBT.

If a team leader only models expertise and success in following the team principles and the DBT manual, however, the team leader can inadvertently set an expectation for perfection. This nondialectical style does not model the vulnerability needed to maintain therapy for the therapist. As mentioned previously, the team can come to believe it is not desirable to share mistakes and ask for help and may even hide the ways in which they are struggling.

At the other pole, some leaders may be skilled in showing vulnerability. They may demonstrate difficulty following the team agreements and be quick to admit to mistakes and ask for help. Doing so models how the team agreements and therapy for the therapist can benefit the team, demonstrates how all team members can show vulnerability, and normalizes the difficulty of following the team agreements. If, however, the leader demonstrates vulnerability nondialectically, without demonstrating skill, expertise, and knowledge, particularly if the team leader is the most experienced individual in the team, the team members may not see the leader as a role model and may not benefit from the leader's expertise and/or experience. Or the team members may learn not to take the team agreements or adherence to the DBT manual seriously, and instead emulate the leader's behavior of admitting to mistakes but not fixing them. Team members may come to believe that it is impossible to follow the agreements or manual. Taken to an extreme, leaders may lose the respect of their teammates for not addressing and resolving problems such as arriving late and incorporating the team's suggestions in sessions.

Synthesizing these two poles is very important in navigating the team leader role. Leaders do need to model following the team agreements, while at the same time exhibit the natural struggle to follow the agreements and to manage inherent challenges. The synthesis is to share mistakes with the team, while handling these mistakes very skillfully by striving to improve at all times, placing themselves on the agenda, taking feedback nondefensively, implementing the team suggestions, and sharing the success with the team. In other words, the leader models skill *and* vulnerability, shows struggle as well as competence. Team members seeing a leader struggle openly, admitting mistakes, and questioning the path forward will emulate this behavior. It is surprisingly helpful for the team to view the leader as one who does not always have the answers. In fact, the team will benefit if the leader is the most fallible in team, while simultaneously modeling absorbing and implementing feedback. This follows the aims of the team (therapy for the therapist, providing the best DBT possible), and sets a standard for team members' behavior that is most effective for the team and clients.

Being a Team Leader versus Being a Team Member

Being a team leader inevitably creates a separation from the rest of the team in certain regards. The team leader is often responsible for monitoring and shaping the form of the program and the team culture. The leader may have more control over certain decisions than other team members, such as the structure of the team, team membership policies, and which clients are assigned to whom. The leader may also (but not necessarily) be more experienced or more trained in DBT and have more opportunity to correct and guide other team members, which again sets up a separation from the other members. In some cases, the team leader will also be liable for the behavior of the team members (e.g., when trainees are operating under the leader's license, or the team leader owns the clinic), which can create strong urges for the leader to correct, monitor, and control team members. The team can benefit greatly from a leader's guidance. A leader who focuses on the big picture, adjusts the course of the team, and maintains the structure of the team and program to enhance team functioning is of great benefit. A leader's experience and mentorship can also be invaluable. At times the leader may exert influence over other team members' behavior, emphasizing the importance of or even demanding change. At its extreme, however, embodying the leadership role in a polarized manner can result in a variety of problems, all relating to difficulties in following the team agreements. First, team members may experience this difference in power and role and behave differently as a result. They may keep certain vulnerabilities hidden or hesitate to challenge the leader. Second, they may reinforce very strong leadership, and as a result become quite passive themselves, relying on the leader to tell them where they need to make changes. Additionally, the leader can end up feeling separate from the team, making it difficult to follow the agreements themselves. For all of these reasons, it is important leaders do not fall into a consultant role where they are the "expert" but not acting as a full member of the team.

While it is true that the team leader may have several qualities that result in a separate role in team, the team leader also functions as a full member of the team, an equal participant. While in team, the leader has the same agreements, the same active seeking of and openness to feedback, the same vulnerabilities as the other members. The leader will need to remain active, fallible, and vulnerable, with a team that treats them equally, with the same support and acceptance, and the same pressure to adhere to the treatment manual. The team will also benefit from a leader who is able to sit back and allow other team members to attend to and solve problems instead of the leader doing so. It will be important for the leader to expect and request that the team questions the leader's decisions, highlights the other pole, makes suggestions, and attends to obstacles that interfere with the leader's fidelity.

Once again, if taken in isolation, acting only as a member of the team can also be problematic. If the team leader fails to shape the team and uphold the agreements of the team, the team culture will likely drift and lose its structure. Team members will not look to the leader as a source of assistance and support. The team leader has an important role in leading the team to maintain its agreements and culture.

The synthesis is for leaders to throw themselves fully into the culture and agreements of the team, while at the same time accepting that their role necessitates some separation. Just as with other dialectics in team, the leader may lean toward one pole in any given moment. This balance may shift across team meetings and across time too. For example, with a team with many trainees, the team leader may emphasize leadership more than membership (e.g., instructing, telling team members what to do), and as the trainees develop and learn, the balance can sway more toward the team leader's membership (e.g., allowing team members to coach each other and not using the leadership role to emphasize what team members need to do). The principles of dialectics and effectiveness can help guide the leader's stance at any given time.

Attending to Team Needs versus Others' Needs

The team leader must balance the team's needs with others' needs, including those of individual team members, clients, and the agency/ treatment setting. A team leader's job is to attend to the team agreements, team culture, team members, and so on. As described above, this is an extremely important position for the health of the DBT team. If, however, the team leader focuses only on the team, other important factors may be neglected. The team leader will discover that the team's needs must be balanced with multiple other demands.

For example, each individual member of the team has needs that may not align with the team at large. At times, an individual team member's needs will even be in direct conflict with the team's needs. For example, when a team member is frustrated with a decision the team leader has made, the team leader may want to make changes to soothe the team member, yet that action may not be best for the team. A provider on our team made a request to get consultation in team on a non-DBT client he was treating. This team member made the argument that this client was increasing his burnout, and getting help would improve his ability to be effective with his DBT clients as well. I (JS) considered this request carefully, and seriously considered approving it because it would help this provider, his client, and his entire caseload. However, this would affect the amount of time other team members would receive in team and change the focus of the team away from DBT. I ultimately decided that the consistency of the team's conceptualization and approach, as well as the importance of other team members' needs, were more important than the individual team member's request. I informed him that he could not bring up this client in team, and suggested he get consultation outside of team from someone with expertise in that particular treatment and client population.

In this example, I chose to protect the team's needs, but leaders may have to make decisions that are not ideal for the team at times. Many team leaders may experience pressure from agency administration or other business considerations to increase funding, cut components of a program, or otherwise create policies that are not in the team's or clients' best interest. The team leader must try to protect the DBT team's principles as much as possible, but needs to also consider that some decisions may harm the business, agency, and/or budget that could result in harm to the team as well. At times, the leader will have to choose a path that is not aligned with team principles, in order to maintain a budget or fulfill an agency policy. For example, an agency may decide to increase the caseload requirement for providers and expect the team leader to enforce the new policy. Ideally, team leaders will use data on the efficacy of DBT in general as well as its effectiveness in this particular setting, along with information pertaining to DBT's cost-effectiveness and the protection from liability that evidence-based treatments provide, to influence agencies and protect the team agreements, but of course this will not always be sufficient. The team leader must synthesize both needs in order to have a healthy financial/administrative environment and to maintain the team.

There may also be tension between the team and a particular client. Recently, a clinician in my (JS) team had a client become very angry and frustrated with her individual therapist. The client called me to register a complaint against her, and the team had a strong desire for me to respond in a certain way. Balancing the needs of both parties did not mean both sides received the exact outcome they wanted, but it did help me make decisions from the most wise position possible. In this case, consultation to the individual therapist (coaching her how to respond) and consultation to the client (coaching the client to use interpersonal skills to speak to her individual therapist) was most effective.

In these dialectical dilemmas, the synthesis will rarely mean appeasing two parties or making a perfect compromise. The leader will have to make difficult decisions based on DBT principles, team agreements, and effectively reaching clinical and administrative goals. Mindfully considering and finding the value in both poles will help the team leader make the most effective decision possible.

Team Leaders Need Support

Being a DBT team leader can be an extremely rewarding and enriching experience. It can also be quite challenging at times! Managing team problems such as interpersonal conflict, drift from the treatment manual, and provider burnout can require skill and energy. We have seen many examples of a struggling leader having a significant impact on team members and, therefore, clients. It makes sense, then, that team leaders will need support, not just for their clinical work, but in their role as team leader.

Remembering the transactional nature of the team and the leader is important here: the team influences the leader just as much as the leader influences the team. The leader may need to request validation, empathy, and reinforcement from the team at times. The team may be unaware of their influence on the leader, such as when they complain about a certain policy or team problem. Leaders can discuss their own struggles with these problems, and ask for validation or problem solving when it is effective to do so.

The leader may also find consulting with other team leaders is useful for particular team problems. For example, one leader sought consultation when her team seemed to repeatedly drift from the DBT manual and expressed frustration when she highlighted the problem. After several attempts, she realized she needed outside help. She contacted another DBT team leader and requested validation, help with problem assessment, and brainstorming for solutions. The consultant had experienced something similar and was able to empathize and provide ideas the team leader had not thought of before. This gave her the morale boost and new ideas that helped move the team forward.

Conclusion

We have seen a wide variety of approaches to team leadership, and we do not see that there is one correct way to do things. Seeking out and rigidly following rules will take the leader far from the team's needs; using mindfulness, assessment, and careful problem solving alongside the team will likely yield the best results. The more a solution is tailored to one's own team, the higher the likelihood of its success. Doing so can create a wonderfully enriching experience for the leader and the team. More on the DBT team leader role can be found in Swales and Dunkley (2019).

IDEAS FOR PRACTICE

These can be practiced by the team leader and/or any other team members.

- Have a team discussion about team leadership, what is going well, and where changes could be made.
- Practice tolerating the distress of not controlling teammates. Mindfully observe the tension generated when a teammate is vulnerable and describes a mistake or misstep in therapy; try validating first and delaying suggestions for change.
- Practice suggesting behavior change to teammates. Practice doing so with individual teammates and with the team at large.
- Discuss and obtain feedback regarding team structure. With the team, problem-solve one structural difficulty the team experiences and implement solutions.
- Do a DEAR MAN with someone in your administration or leadership (if relevant) for a change that would benefit the team.
- Practice seeing the team from an administrator's point of view.
- Write out the team leader's dialectical dilemmas and which pole(s), if any, you tend to lean toward.
- Practice asking the team for support for your challenges in fulfilling leadership tasks.
- Identify a source of support outside the team for the challenges in fulfilling leadership tasks.

The Structure of the DBT Team
The Agenda

With roles in place, it's time to start running the team! Keeping in mind the main job of the team is to facilitate adherent DBT, via increasing each member's capability and motivation, setting a structure for team time can maximize these functions and remove obstacles to adhering to the DBT manual. This chapter provides a basic structure for the team meeting that can be used as a guide. This structure can help maintain the focus on therapy for the therapist and the other agreements listed in Chapter 1.

The team can set the agenda verbally, with members calling out items to the meeting leader, and the meeting leader writing the items on the agenda at the start of the meeting. However, this method takes up team time; an alternative is to have members write their name on a written agenda as they walk in, before mindfulness practice, either on paper or on a whiteboard. See Handouts 9 and 10 for two sample written agendas with different formats; teams can experiment with these and develop a format that works best for them. Time allotted to agenda items will depend on the length of the team meeting and the needs of each member; the written agendas provided are based on 90- to 120-minute team meetings.

When team members add themselves to the agenda, it is helpful to indicate how urgent their items are. The DBT treatment hierarchy, distress, and time sensitivity guide prioritization. Prioritization of agenda items is discussed further below. Some teams also find it helpful for members to give an estimated amount of time needed.

Topics for the Agenda

In order to provide therapy for the therapist, members of the team place *themselves* on the agenda, instead of a client. Rather than focusing on a client's behavior and how to change the client, in DBT team the focus is placed on the team member's behavior. Because providers place themselves on the agenda, rather than specific clients, each member will have only one turn on the agenda. There is no need to put oneself on the agenda multiple times for multiple clients; each team member on the agenda will have one turn to discuss one or more obstacles to clinical care.

For example, in a non-DBT team, providers might say they need help because their client is not working hard enough in therapy. Placing oneself on the agenda would change this language slightly; the team member might instead request, "I am frustrated, my client is not following through with homework. I could use some skills for regulating my frustration, and I'd also like to brainstorm strategies I can use to increase homework completion." Rather than saying, "My client is calling too much," putting oneself on the agenda would translate this to: "I'm noticing my limits are getting stretched by the number of calls I'm receiving. I am dreading my phone ringing. I need help with two things: first, I'd like to talk about my limits and that I'm really tired of stretching them for this client, and second, I would like to role-play telling my client I want to change the way our phone calls go." When DBT providers are not sure what they need, they might say, "I'm going to need some help! I'm really emotional about this client but I don't understand why or what to do." Simple changes in language can help enhance therapy for the therapist; instead of saying, "My client is frustrating!," which places the focus on the client, the provider can say, "I feel frustrated by my client," which moves the focus onto the team member.

What goes on the agenda, exactly? One can place any item on the agenda that helps address the DBT provider's obstacles to adherent, effective treatment. These may include:

- A skills deficit (e.g., not knowing how to deliver a certain intervention or strategy, such as stimulus control, devil's advocate, or exposure).
- A lack of knowledge (e.g., not knowing what the evidence-based treatment for insomnia is).

- A life circumstance that is affecting quality of care (e.g., when a therapist is getting a divorce, that can make it difficult to work with a client getting a divorce).

- A team member's own emotion (e.g., experiencing intense fear with a client can make it difficult to make effective decisions).

- Decreased motivation to follow the manual or otherwise engage in the DBT team and treatment (e.g., feeling burned out, having urges to do something other than the treatment).

- One's own or a team member's behavior that interferes with the team's functioning (e.g., judgments in team).

Note that one *can* get traditional clinical consultation from the team, in which the team helps decide how to respond to a particular clinical problem. But this type of conversation is not the main emphasis; it only becomes the team strategy when lack of knowledge is interfering with providing the best care possible.

When the problem is a skills or knowledge deficit, the team will offer specific, concrete information (e.g., didactics on particular disorders, populations, or research) and suggestions (e.g., obtaining a particular manual or other source of information, consulting with an expert in that treatment, or referring the client to a specialist in that area). For example, a team member may ask the team for information regarding a particular cultural issue, where to refer a client for a medication problem, or which manual to use to treat a specific problem. The team may also ask that team member to rehearse a new skill in team, or conduct a chain analysis of a behavior in session. Not all problems raised will be emotional or personal; the focus remains on addressing whatever obstacles interfere with adherent DBT.

At times, a team member might think, "There's no way I'm talking about this in team!" Some problems or emotions may feel too personal to share in team. DBT team members do not need to share every detail of their personal lives (limits are important here!), and in fact, most personal problems do not come up in team. Only those personal problems that interfere with providing effective DBT need to be addressed. If the problem is interfering and the team member does not want to discuss it in team, that team member will need to acknowledge the problem but does not need to provide details. The team will simply need some reassurance that the problem is being dealt with, such that treatment will not be negatively impacted. This may be as simple as informing the team that there are problems in one's personal life and one is working on solutions with one's own therapist outside of team. If a team member is unwilling to discuss the problem and it continues to have an impact on the team or client(s), the leader may need to intervene; starting with an individual meeting will likely be most effective in this case. And some problems may be too large for the team, or outside of the team's area of expertise. This topic is addressed further in Chapter 5.

Problems with the team's healthy functioning also belong on the agenda. When a team member brings up a problem with team function-ing, it is important to be mindful, avoid defensiveness, and reinforce their willingness to discuss the topic openly. It can be harmful to let problems in the team fester; they need to be talked about, even if it feels much easier to avoid the problem and pretend that nothing has happened (this would be an elephant in the room!). Addressing problems in team is dis-cussed further in Chapter 6.

There is, of course, a dialectic in addressing team problems. On the one hand, DBT places high value on being direct and open about one's challenges in team; on the other hand, not all problems must be discussed. The most effective balance of acceptance and change can be determined using skills such as Wise Mind, Radical Acceptance, and Effectiveness. Some avoidance will be necessary to keep the team mov-ing forward; if the team tries to address every challenging moment in team, team members will not be able to provide the best care for cli-ents. Team members can ask themselves, "Will talking about this issue, or continuing to talk about this issue, be in the best interest of my client and my team?" Remaining focused on the goal of adherent DBT, and only addressing problems that interfere with that goal, can help the team decide when and if to address such difficulties or to let them slide in order to address higher priority topics.

Topics to Exclude from the Clinical Agenda

Topics that do not facilitate therapy for the therapist will be better addressed outside of DBT team time, as they take away time from the team's goal of enhancing clinical care. There are a few topics that often are best addressed outside of team. Once again, these are principles and should not be followed rigidly or mindlessly; each team can make their own decisions about how to handle these topics. Excluded topics may include:

- Administrative and business items.
- Didactics/training topics.
- Intervening with a teammate on behalf of a client (most of the time).
- Certain ethical issues and other sensitive topics.
- Listing problems for the sake of listing problems.

Administrative and Business Items

Administrative and business items, such as finances, policies, marketing, and program development, do not fit with the team's purpose and aims, and therefore should be discussed at a separate time (although brief announcements may be useful).

Didactics/Training Topics

A team may focus on didactics and training early in its development, but as the team evolves into a fully formed DBT team, didactics and training will also take place outside of the team meeting, or in a distinct period of time in team (e.g., some teams reserve the last 30 minutes of team for training, journal articles, and so on; this part of the meeting is purposefully not focused on therapy for the therapist). The principle here is to make sure that team time is focused on therapy for the therapist; these types of agenda items do not involve therapy for the therapist, and should be addressed separately. Teams may find some overlap between clinical and administrative issues (e.g., asking for coverage while a team member is out of town); teams can mindfully decide if these types of topics are best addressed during team or in another setting.

Intervening with a Teammate on Behalf of a Client (Most of the Time)

Team members will likely find it helpful to inform each other of issues with a shared client. The DBT team provides the opportunity to update each other and come to a shared formulation and treatment plan, particularly when more than one team member interacts with the client. However, in such cases, teams will need to be mindful of the consultation to the client and environmental intervention strategies (Linehan, 1993). These strategies are dialectical in nature; they balance providing consultation to clients, so they can skillfully intervene upon the environment themselves, with being the change agent for clients. This dialectic comes up regularly in team; team members may come to a team meeting wanting to change another member of the team or solve a problem on behalf of a client. For example, a skills leader may learn that a client is upset with their individual therapist for being judgmental in their last session, and that skills leader may want to correct the individual therapist in team to help the client. Whenever possible, members of the team will try to coach clients to handle the situation themselves (in this example, coach the client to speak to the individual therapist directly, and offer skills and suggestions for how the client can navigate that situation), to provide the client the opportunity to learn to manage the situations themselves.

It will be important that the team does not rigidly avoid environmental intervention, however. There are times when it will be worth foregoing the learning opportunity and the provider will choose an environmental intervention with another member of the team. For example, when a client has significant risk or other urgent problems, or is simply exhausted, it may be worth quickly intervening with another provider on behalf of the client, so the client can focus on their highest-priority targets. While most often team members will strive to avoid environmental interventions, it is helpful to consider the context and then mindfully decide which strategy will be most beneficial.

Focusing on consultation to the client and environmental intervention does not preclude team members from informing each other that a problem exists with a particular client. Teams may discuss client difficulties, brainstorm solutions, and even alert each other when a client will be addressing a problem with another team member; the main principle here is to provide the client with as many learning opportunities as possible. Team members can help weigh the pros and cons of these strategies as needed.

Certain Ethical Issues and Other Sensitive Topics

With effective development of the DBT team culture, there will be significantly less need to censor oneself and less fear of being too direct.

However, there are a few topics that may be too sensitive to discuss in a team format, at least for some members. If a member of the team is accused of unethical behavior, they may prefer to hold this discussion outside of the team, perhaps with the team leader. Such a topic is highly sensitive and could have significant impact on one's career and reputation and thus should be handled cautiously. At some point this topic may come back to team, but it will likely be unhelpful if the team member is forced to discuss it first in the team setting. Other topics that are less likely to be discussed in team might include a team member's legal situation (if involved in a legal situation regarding one's own client, it is wise to obtain legal counsel regarding how much and when to talk to the team), or employment status, salary, or other employment-related topics.

Teams should also avoid *forcing* a team member to discuss a sensitive topic; if a team member is reluctant to discuss a problem that is affecting clinical care, the team leader may intervene outside of team to help the team member figure out how to move forward. The team leader and at some point the team as a whole can help balance this team member's limits, the client's needs, and the team's functioning.

Listing Problems for the Sake of Listing Problems

Interpersonal conflict between team members could interfere with team functioning and client care; in such cases the conflict can be addressed in or out of team but it must be addressed. These conflicts might include one team member experiencing invalidation from another teammate or feeling slighted by a comment made in team. On the other hand, as mentioned above, the DBT team is not the time to list all of the problems one has with another team member; only those issues that impact fidelity to the treatment and team agreements are discussed in team. For example, the team may become frustrated by one member's intense responses to topics in team; teammates can mindfully decide whether this is "just the way they are," and tolerate their own irritation, or if these reactions indeed interfere with client care or team functioning and need to be addressed. We have seen team members bring up multiple annoyances with other team members, even though they do not affect client care; in such cases, the team gets bogged down in the interpersonal issues and drifts away from focusing on providing DBT. Acceptance and other skills can be used to tolerate frustrations with other team members. Similarly, this is not a time for team members to list all of their own personal problem, unless directly related to their clinical work; providers may want to seek out their own therapy in this case. Agenda items are thoughtfully placed on the agenda only when they are impacting client care (motivation, capability) and/or team functioning.

A Structure for DBT Team Meetings

We have found the structure below to be extremely useful for many teams. Using this exact agenda is not essential (we are, once again, relying on principles, not rules). There is no particular order for these topics, either, although certain items may be more effective if they fall earlier in the team (e.g., mindfulness first, reminders about the agenda should come before moving through the agenda). The first seven items are more commonly used in DBT teams, and the remaining items are examples of creative additions some teams use. As long as therapy for the therapist occurs and the needs of the team are addressed, teams have great flexibility in how they set up the team meeting.

DBT team meetings often include the following agenda items:

- Mindfulness
- Read agreement(s)
- Read last meeting's notes
- Agenda reminders
- Move through the agenda
- Share effective behaviors
- Close the team meeting
- Team member check-ins
- Team member of the week
- Coordination of care
- Observer questions

Mindfulness

We recommend that every team begins their meeting each week with a mindfulness practice. This can consist of either silent meditation or an exercise. Some teams use this time as an opportunity to practice the mindfulness exercise that will be taught in skills group that week; others have team members engage in their own individual practice as they wish. After mindfulness, members very briefly describe their experience. Mindfulness practice should take approximately 5 minutes, with comments taking no more than another 5 minutes. This is a useful way to reinforce the importance of mindfulness in the treatment, to provide time for practice, and to focus team members' attention on the team meeting.

Read Agreement(s)

The meeting leader chooses one team agreement from the core DBT team agreements (see Chapter 1 and Handout 1) to read aloud. Teams may add other reminders at this time, as well, such as an assumption about clients and/or therapy, and/or one of the observer agreements. Teams may also add other team agreements discussed in Chapter 1 to this list, if the team needs particular reminders to function well. This portion of team is very brief and serves as a reminder regarding the culture of the team.

Read Last Meeting's Notes

If the team takes notes in each meeting, the notes from the previous meeting can be read or displayed. This serves to help team members remember what was agreed upon in the previous meeting. It is very easy to lose track of ongoing problems or plans without reviewing previous notes. If one of the team members realizes they forgot to follow up on something, they can add it to the current agenda. This is also a useful tool if a teammate is avoiding certain topics—the team can make sure that avoidance is blocked!

Agenda Reminders

Teams often find it useful to prompt team members on certain topics, to be sure they place it on the agenda. These reminders can be generated by the team to address any topics the team would find helpful. The meeting leader can ask, "Does anyone have the following? If so, do you want to add yourself to the agenda?" For example:

- A client who is at higher risk for suicide this week?
- A client who is at risk of missing four sessions in a row?

- A need for back-up coverage for travel?
- Paperwork requirements that are out of date?
- A client who is engaging in increasingly ineffective behaviors?
- A client near the end of the treatment agreement period? (This serves as a reminder for a discussion of termination, related termination paperwork/assessments, or a renewal of the treatment agreement.)
- A team member who spent a lot of time phone coaching this week? (The team can help assess whether any problematic behaviors are being reinforced.)
- A team member who was late; is a chain analysis needed?

Team members are not required to discuss these items, but if there are obstacles to maintaining fidelity to the treatment manual, these prompts serve to remind team members to place themselves on the agenda if needed. It is extremely easy for busy DBT providers to forget certain agenda items, and these reminders can help jog their memories.

Move through the Agenda

Once all of the reminders are given and the agenda is set, the meeting leader then guides the team through the agenda. In order to maintain the focus on the provider rather than on the client, and help the team meet the provider's needs, when it is their turn, each team member makes a specific request from the team. The provider chooses from a list of requests, which serves to focus both the team member and the team, and lends efficiency and precision to the team's discussion. Many teams use the following list when a team member requests help from the team:*

1. "I'd like help assessing a particular problem, and/or . . . "
2. "Help generating solutions for a particular problem, and/or . . . "
3. "Help empathizing with a client, and/or . . . "
4. "Validation from the team."

---

*Adapted with permission from Marsha M. Linehan, unpublished, University of Washington Behavioral Research and Therapy Clinics.

To these four basic requests, teams may add other categories, such as "I need help with burnout" or "I need help figuring out what I need." Teams can feel free to adjust this list as it benefits the team; the main principle is that team members state what they need, to avoid the team spending time solving problems the provider has already solved or miss opportunities for much needed validation. Team members can state their request aloud at the start of their consultation time, and/or write it on the agenda.

I (JS) recently had a member of our team describe a difficult situation in which a client had high suicidal urges and had purchased a gun. The team, feeling frightened and concerned, immediately started problem solving how to get rid of the gun. The provider actually needed help building empathy, not problem solving. She had to stop the team and clarify her request; she already had successfully implemented a solution for getting rid of the gun, so time spent on the issue of removing the gun was not helpful. The team then refocused on what she did need: rebuilding empathy when she had intense frustration and fear. This is a situation where the team member, the observer, or any other team member can highlight that the team is not focusing on what their teammate needs.

Many team members just want to "vent," or tell the team a detailed account of what has happened and how awful it was. This may actually be exactly what is needed in the moment: to describe everything, express emotion, and receive validation. In this case, one can request validation from the team. However, venting is not always helpful; it can lead to an increase in judgments, move the team away from behavioral specificity, and obscure the problem. It is important to mindfully consider what is most useful, and for the team to provide feedback. The therapist might also ask for both: "I'd love a little validation, then I'm going to need some help problem solving." Again, mindfully requesting help in a specific area, and having everyone on the team stay alert to whether the conversation is on-topic and productive (i.e., beneficial to the client, addressing the team member's needs) is very important.

Prioritization

When team members put themselves on the agenda, they also note their own priority. Teams use the DBT hierarchy (Linehan, 1993) to determine how urgent items are (a provider dealing with life-threatening behavior would take priority over providers dealing with therapy-interfering or quality-of-life behaviors), as well as how distressed the team member feels about the situation, and how time-sensitive the topic is (e.g., whether consultation is needed before a session later in the day). In our experience, team members are typically able to determine if they must take a turn in team, or if it can wait until the next team or for informal consultation during the week. This prioritization can be done verbally, with the leader documenting who needs to go first and who can wait, or the urgency can be rated on a written agenda. (Our teams follow the format of the diary card: a 5 rating means "I must have time in team today," while a 1 means "If we run out of time it's OK to skip me today.")

If a team member only uses their own distress as a means to rate their priority, teams may end up with one person dominating the team time to the exclusion of other team members who are dealing with high-risk situations but whose emotions are less intense. Teams will want to be sure certain providers or topics are not excluded inadvertently; using the hierarchy and time sensitivity, as well as individual distress, as guidelines will help teams prioritize effectively.

High-priority items we would rate as a 5 might include:

"I need validation today because I'm frustrated and am seeing the client again this week." (time sensitive)

"I need help assessing my client's suicide risk, I am struggling and the risk is high." (life-threatening behavior that needs immediate intervention)

"I need help with a distressing therapy-interfering behavior." (therapy-interfering behavior and high provider distress)

"I have a phone call later today with the client and her psychiatrist and need help knowing how to manage the call." (not high risk, but time sensitive)

"My client is quickly approaching four misses." (therapy-interfering behavior and time sensitive)

"I have so much going on in my life that I worry that my own intense emotions will interfere with effective therapy for everyone." (high provider distress)

These all warrant a high rating, which communicates to the meeting leader that a team member needs time in team today.

Medium-priority items we would rate as a 3 or 4 might include:

"I'm frustrated with my client, but I at least know what to do in my next session."

"I am struggling with irreverence with a few clients, but it's not urgent."

"I could use some ideas for solutions because the plan for my client's work problems has not been helpful."

"I am noticing I'm more irritable with one of my clients. I have a plan for now but I will need some team help."

"My client has an anniversary coming up that will cause distress. It's not this week, but I'd like to review our plan with the team in the next 2 weeks."

These items will most likely get covered in the current team meeting, but the medium rating allows for higher priority items to go first. If the provider does not get a turn in this meeting, they can increase the priority rating in the next team meeting.

Finally, lowest-priority items, rated 1 or 2, might include:

"I need help identifying resources for my client for employment in the next few weeks."

"I have maternity leave coming up in 2 months and would like to talk about certain clients' distress regarding my leave."

" I am judging a client a lot and need help bringing the judgments down, but I don't see the client again for 2 weeks."

By rating these items as low priority, the provider is communicating that it is perfectly fine for these items to wait another week if necessary; the provider can then give them a higher rating in an upcoming team meeting as they become more urgent.

The meeting leader uses the prioritization indicated by team members to choose who will speak first. The individual who indicated the highest priority will go first; if there are several high-priority items, the leader will simply start at the top and work their way down the list. As mentioned above, a team may prefer to have providers estimate how much time they will need. This helps the meeting leader plan the team and know how tightly the team needs to stick to the agenda, or whether certain members can be given extra time if requested. The meeting leader will watch the clock and give each team member the amount of time asked for. If more time is still needed after the time is up, the team will briefly discuss whether something else on the agenda can be postponed in order to afford this individual more time, the individual needs to get consultation outside of team in order to complete the conversation, or the matter can be postponed until the following team meeting.

After the team member describes the situation and what is needed, the team will do its best to meet that need (by gathering more information, validating, problem solving, etc.), and/or suggest to the team member that something other than what was asked for might prove useful (e.g., suggest more assessment is needed prior to providing requested solutions). The team member can give feedback to the team regarding what was helpful, such as, "You aren't focused on the right spot!," which allows the team to adjust as needed, or the team can clarify what is needed (e.g., ask for more information before providing the requested coaching, or suggest the team member needs to build empathy before problem solving). As the team moves in to try to help their teammate, the observer and all members will be alert for signs that the team is straying from the topic at hand and will highlight this digression so the team may make corrections.

The team member requesting help does *not* need to feel obligated to use every solution or suggestion generated by the team. The team will trust that their teammate has sufficient skill and knowledge about the client to choose the best possible course of action (of course, a supervisor or primary investigator may require certain responses). If the team offers solutions that are not useful, the provider can either say, "Thanks, I've already tried that," very briefly and redirect the team, or ask for more ideas from the team. Spending a great deal of time turning down every solution the team offers can waste time and cause more tension in team. This may be a sign that the team doesn't fully understand the problem, or is not trusting the idea that their teammate has implemented a solution thoroughly enough, or is getting distracted by an emotional topic (such as a gun in the above example). To avoid an "elephant in the room," it will be important to discuss these kinds of concerns directly and openly.

Consultation will continue for nearly all the remaining team time.

The leader will work down the priority list, such that each member, or nearly every member, who requested team time will receive a turn.

Share Effective Behaviors

We have found it is very helpful to share effective behaviors, of our own and of our clients, in team. Particularly when team members are experiencing high stress or high-risk clinical situations, hearing examples of the treatment working well and getting feedback that their previous suggestions proved fruitful can be a meaningful reminder of why everyone in the team is doing this hard work. Discussing successes is a powerful motivator for many providers, and will contribute to team morale and dedication significantly. Doing so at the end of the team meeting can set an optimistic tone for the coming week.

Close the Team Meeting

The meeting leader then indicates it is time to end the team meeting. This may be done by simply announcing the time or by ringing a mindfulness bell. The team should end on time even if not all agenda items were covered; team members will become more skilled over time at estimating the time needed for various problems and moving through an agenda in a more timely manner. While closing the team meeting may only take 1 second, it can be important, particularly if certain team members tend to continue speaking beyond the scheduled time, or team members walk out while others are still talking. Ringing the bell or otherwise alerting team members that they have reached the end of the scheduled time allows for the meeting to end at a predictable time without creating tension or frustration.

The above seven items are fairly standard in most DBT teams. As mentioned above, teams can adapt the agenda as needed, adding or eliminating items if it helps the team. Below are some additional suggestions for team agendas.

Team Member Check-Ins

In our (JS) team, we realized it was difficult to be vulnerable with each other when we were not aware of the latest events in each other's lives. We found it very useful to add time to the agenda for "team member check-ins." We have found that other teams enjoy this kind of time as well. During this time, team members briefly (i.e., approximately 1 minute per person) describe any events from the past week that they wish to share, including emotional, silly, and nonconsequential events. For example, someone might share recent family stressors such as a child's illness, or accomplishments, or what movie they saw the previous weekend. Members also share their level of burnout and general distress, to alert the team if they are struggling for any reason. This check-in is kept brief; any items requiring team attention can be placed on the agenda. We have found these check-ins to be very helpful in enhancing a feeling of closeness; however, this can take up more time than some teams can afford.

Team Member of the Week

If a team chooses to include a "team member of the week" in the agenda, the meeting leader will typically begin the clinical agenda with this segment. Described in Chapter 2, this segment of a team meeting provides a mechanism for each team member to bring up less acute, yet important, obstacles to effective treatment. This time allows topics that might not otherwise rise to the highest priority to be addressed with more forethought and preparation. This often includes a role play, video, and/or case formulation. Team members each state what they need from the list above (e.g., "I need help with problem solving") before starting. The team member of the week typically takes 15 minutes. It is a rotating assignment, rather than one based on acuity. A list of team members of the week and dates can be posted in advance.

Coordination of Care

Teams may also choose to devote some team time to coordination of care, if multiple team members are involved with the same client. For example, if there is a psychiatrist on the team, it can be very useful to give the psychiatrist a short period of time to inform the team of which clients were seen in the past week, briefly review any issues that need discussion, and list the clients who will be seen in the coming week. Skills trainers may also use this time to inform individual therapists and other team members which skills were taught in the past week, what homework was assigned, and what will be taught in the coming week.

This portion of team does not directly function as therapy for the therapist (although it may also result in team members putting themselves
on the agenda to get help with particular problems that have arisen),
but it provides the individual therapist with information necessary to
coordinate care. While in traditional teams this coordination of care is
the main focus of the team, in the DBT team this is kept brief; if the
team spends too much time updating, the therapy for the therapist function can be lost. The meeting leader must be mindful of time and move
the team quickly to the main agenda items (therapy for the therapist).
We find it helpful to put a limit on the amount of time spent, such as
10 minutes, for this item; it may also be helpful to place it toward the
end of the agenda to make sure it does not interfere with therapy for the
therapist. Other teams simply communicate by e-mail so updating does
not take up any team time.

Observer Questions

Our (JS) team began leaving time (5 minutes) at the end of team meeting for the observer to read all of the observer reminders (briefly), asking the team if those behaviors occurred during team. We made this
change with the goal of increasing the salience of the reminders. This
also promotes a situation in which *all* members observe and comment
on the team culture rather than relying solely on the observer. Team
members briefly discuss each observer reminder (e.g., "Was there a team
member who did not speak during team?"; "Did anyone make judgmental
or noncompassionate statements today?"), out themselves as needed ("I
think I was judgmental when I talked about my client."), reinforce each
other for effective behavior, and suggest brief solutions for areas where
the team strayed from the agreements. This discussion is nonjudgmental
and focused on promoting healthy team culture. If one of the questions
generates a more lengthy discussion, it can be placed on the agenda for
the next team meeting.

Certain teams may have a specific purpose or aim that may require
alterations to the above agenda. For example, a DBT team in an inpatient, residential, or intensive outpatient setting may meet more frequently (often daily), and have a wider variety of staff roles attending.
With this type of team, the principles of the DBT team will remain
the same, but the members may add certain components, such as time

to coordinate with milieu staff or to discuss discharge plans. Another example is a research team, in which the team is providing treatment as part of a research study. Once again, certain adjustments may be made, such that the research protocol is incorporated into the team meeting. For example, the agenda reminders might include monitoring whether team members are following the research protocol, collecting proper assessments, and so on. Research teams may also change the hierarchy of the team meeting, such that the focus of research (e.g., substance use, depression) is considered as high a priority as life-threatening behavior is in standard DBT. Training teams may also require certain modifications. In a training team, typically the team leader has extensive DBT experience, and some or all of the other team members have significantly less experience. This type of team might require the leader to be more directive and active than the other members. The team leader or other experienced members must remain aware of shaping newer members into becoming active members of the team, coaching and reinforcing effective team behaviors such as providing the leader with feedback and highlighting a dialectic, even when the newer members are less experienced and knowledgeable. Such teams run the risk of team members relying on the experienced member for answers, and the team leader intervening for the entire team, which is not consistent with the DBT team agreements. The experienced members will need to remain continuously focused on shaping the team into implementing the DBT team agreements.

Example 1

In Figure 4.1, we provide an example of Handout 9 to illustrate how the team might move through a DBT team agenda. Each team member determined their own priority rating and requested an amount of time to discuss their agenda item.

In this case, if the team meeting were 90 minutes long, the meeting leader would spend approximately 20 minutes conducting mindfulness, reading an agreement, briefly reviewing the previous team meeting's notes, reading the agenda reminders, and asking group leaders to update the team on skills taught in the previous skills groups. The meeting leader would then tell team member of the week, CH, to begin the "team member of the week" portion of the agenda, 15 minutes set aside

FIGURE 4.1. DBT team meeting agenda: Example 1.

Team member indicates a need for one or more of the following when speaking to the team:

(1) Validation from the team

(2) Help increasing empathy toward client

(3) Help improving assessment with client

(4) Problem-solving suggestions

Check box when topic has been discussed/completed.

❑ Mindfulness
❑ Read agreement
❑ Review last week's notes
❑ Reminders to place on the agenda if more help is needed:
  • Who is treating someone at high risk for imminent suicide?
  • Who is treating a potential four-misses person?
  • Who is going out of town?
  • Who has out-of-date paperwork?
  • Who is treating someone who is doing worse?
  • Who has a client coming to the end of the treatment agreement?
  • Who spent a lot of time on the phone this week?
  • Was anyone late to team today?
❑ Group updates (which skill was taught, homework assigned, upcoming skill)
❑ Team member of the week: _____CH_____

15 minutes spent on one of the following: (1) role play, (2) viewing video, (3) presenting case formulation

PRIORITIZATION:
High priority (e.g., life-threatening behavior, high team member distress, time-sensitive topics, important team-interfering behaviors)
Team member initials:

❑ _DD (10 minutes)_____	❑ _ST (15 minutes)_____
❑ _AL (5 minutes)_____	❑ _____

Medium priority (e.g., topics that are important but not time sensitive, it's OK if we run out of time today)

❑ _AP (5 minutes)_____	❑ _____
❑ _JT (1 minute)_____	❑ _____

Low priority (e.g., topics that can wait; there is a fair chance that these topics may get skipped today)

❑ _LL (10 minutes)_____	❑ _____
❑ _____	❑ _____

Other:
❑ Effective client or team member behaviors/progress _____
❑ Ring bell to end meeting

for showing a video, conducting role plays, and/or discussing a case formulation. CH provides the team with a specific request (e.g., validation, empathy, assessment, and/or problem solving), and the team tries to meet those needs. In this case, CH requests problem solving for a pattern in which therapy often loses its movement, speed, and flow. CH shows a video clip of a session to illustrate this problem. The team assesses, offers several suggestions, and CH rehearses with a teammate how to implement one particular solution (irreverence) for the next session with this client. The meeting leader alerts CH that time is almost up; the team then wraps up that discussion briefly.

The meeting leader then moves to DD, who also states what is needed, then uses 10 minutes to orient the team and obtain consultation. In this case, DD requests help with empathy and assessment. DD says one particular client has been highly suicidal lately. They had made a plan in session, then the client did not follow the plan, which resulted in a high-risk situation. DD expresses frustration and fear that the client had not utilized their skills plan. The team first validates these emotions, then moves on to DD's request: regaining empathy for this client, which was lost when the provider became frustrated, and identifying what variables DD missed, to explain why the plan did not work. The team focuses on building compassion for this client, reminding their teammate how difficult the situation was and how it makes sense the client could not follow the plan in a moment of high distress. They then review DD's chain analysis of this moment and offer suggestions for additional areas to assess and problem-solve. Meanwhile, DD can give feedback as to when the team is on track, and when the team digresses from DD's needs. The meeting leader allows about 10 minutes for this discussion; if this is not sufficient time, the team can discuss whether to add more time and/or address this further outside of team.

The meeting leader proceeds through AL and ST, who are also high priority, then moves on to AP and JT, who are medium priority. Assuming the meeting leader is able to stick to the times suggested, the team will have enough time to get through the low-priority agenda item (LL) too; if the team has run overtime at certain points, LL may need to wait until the next team meeting. The meeting leader then asks if anyone wants to share their own or clients' effective behaviors and rings the bell to close the team meeting. While the meeting leader is proceeding through the agenda in this manner, the observer and the entire team work to maintain the team agreements; offer extensive validation, caring, and humor; and help each teammate obtain what is needed to move treatment forward.

Example 2

The second example, in Figure 4.2, utilizes the second agenda form, which offers more structure and illustrates variation on the agenda items. (This agenda adds a reminder to write the skills taught that week on the whiteboard and time for the following additional activities: a chain analysis for a late team member, team member check-in, coordination of care, and a brief discussion of observer questions.) In this particular example, the team has 2 hours to get through the agenda, so there is extra time to add items that were not included in Example 1. This agenda form also offers more options in terms of what team members might request from the team. In addition to the standard requests (validation, empathy, assessment, problem solving), team members can also indicate on the agenda that they are burned out, they have a brief update for the team, they don't know what they need and could use help figuring it out, or they have a brief announcement.

In this team, the opening agenda items (mindfulness, read an agreement, review notes, read reminders) take about 20 minutes. This team then allots 15 minutes for "team member check-in," which allows time for each team member to briefly update the team on events from the past week. The meeting leader will then tell the team member of the week, OL, that it is their turn. In this case, OL requested help with assessment. OL describes the situation or pattern, and the team primarily focuses on improving OL's assessment of the problem. Next, the team briefly conducts a chain analysis for one late member. The meeting leader then moves through the other individuals on the agenda, calling on the highest-priority team members first (SG, AT, KI), and then the medium-priority member (JT). MM had a brief announcement that, due to its low rating, may get delayed to the next team meeting. The meeting leader saves time for brief coordination of care (e.g., the psychopharmacologist can tell team members who had appointments in the past week), and for the observer to quickly read all of the observer agreements so that the team can identify any problems with maintaining the agreements in team that day (these may be briefly highlighted or discussed at greater length in a subsequent team meeting). The meeting leader closes the meeting by

FIGURE 4.2. DBT team meeting agenda: Example 2.

Date: _____ Leader: _____

Check box when topic has been discussed/completed.

❑ Mindfulness (10 minutes)

❑ Read agreement

❑ Review last week's notes

❑ Skills update on whiteboard

❑ REMINDERS: if you need help with the following, please put on the agenda:

✓ A client who is at a higher risk for suicide?
✓ A client who is at risk of missing four sessions in a row?
✓ A need for back-up coverage for travel?
✓ Paperwork requirements that are out of date?
✓ A client who is engaging in increasingly ineffective behaviors?
✓ A client near the end of the treatment period?
✓ Spent a lot of time phone coaching this week?
✓ Was anyone late to team today?

Place your initials on the agenda. (Remember to put the *team member* on the agenda.)

Check box for what you need today. Indicate priority and minutes needed.

Number of minutes requested	Priority: 1–5 (5 = highest)	Team member initials	I need help with ASSESSMENT	I need help with PROBLEM SOLVING	I need help building EMPATHY for my client	I need VALIDATION	I am BURNED OUT (please define for team)	I have an UPDATE	I DON'T KNOW what I need, but I need HELP!	I have an ANNOUNCEMENT
15	5	Team member check-in								
15	5	Team member of the week: OL	✓							
5	5	Chain analysis for late member								
20	3	JT		✓						
2	1	MM								✓
15	5	SG	✓	✓						
3	5	AT						✓		
10	5	KI							✓	
5	5	Coordination of care								
5	5	Observer questions								
5	5	Effective behavior								
		Close								

inviting team members to share effective behaviors, then formally ends the meeting on time by ringing the bell.

These examples will hopefully highlight the way in which teams start with the basic structure discussed in this chapter, then can adapt and add structure that helps that particular team to meet its needs. Teams can take the forms offered here and tailor them strategically, to help them maximize the effectiveness of their interventions and address any issues unique to that team.

Conclusion

This chapter provides structure for DBT team flow. The structure of any given team does not need to match our suggested forms exactly; mindfully creating and maintaining a structure that meets the team's needs will increase the team's efficiency immensely, leaving more time for discussion of important consultation items. This structure also allows the team to address problems in its functioning head-on. Everyone is given license to bring up and address these issues and will remain vigilant for opportunities to reinforce such behavior. Of course, obstacles will arise, including team members' emotions, interpersonal conflicts, and difficult clinical situations. Some of these problems and potential solutions are addressed in Chapter 6. Problems will be difficult to address if these basic building blocks are not in place. This structure, along with commitment, team roles, and the other elements discussed in this book, form the backbone of a well-running team.

IDEAS FOR PRACTICE

■ Follow the structure described in this chapter exactly for four team meetings. Then review and identify how the structure might be tailored to your own team.

■ Practice identifying what is needed before putting yourself on the agenda. Overtly say, "I am placing myself on the agenda, and I need. . . . " Give each other feedback about the clarity and accuracy of that request.

■ Practice ending a conversation at the end of the allotted time, even if you feel the conversation is not yet complete.

■ Have a team discussion about mindfulness, and how to ensure that there is regular time for mindfulness practice.

- Have a team discussion about which reminders the team would like to hear read aloud, and tailor the meeting leader agreement reminder and observer reminder lists accordingly.
- Have a team discussion about the overall structure of the team, and whether tailoring might be helpful. Experiment with different agenda formats and discuss which are most helpful.

Therapy for the Therapist

As mentioned in previous chapters, an important distinction between traditional treatment teams and the DBT team is DBT's focus on the team member. DBT aims to provide *therapy for the therapist,* rather than discuss clients per se. As we have said previously, the term "therapist" in this context refers to any member of the DBT team (not just to the individual therapist). In the DBT team, each member seeks support, compassion, and help with any obstacles to providing adherent, effective treatment for their DBT clients, and the team helps by validating and solving problems. Therefore, in team, team members place themselves, not their clients, on the agenda, with an explicit request for what type of help they need from the team (validation, empathy, assessment, and/or problem solving; see Chapter 4), in order to guide the team in providing the most effective consultation.

Obstacles to effective DBT might include a variety of issues, such as a lack of knowledge or skill, burnout, intense emotions, or personal difficulties. Thankfully, most of the time meeting a team member's request for help will be quite simple; they may only need some kind words, information, a brief list of skills to offer a client, a reference, or a simple explanation of an agency policy. But other times the situation may be quite complex, such as when the provider's and/or client's emotions inhibit treatment progress. Regardless of the topic, DBT teams implement DBT with each other; the same DBT strategies and skills that are used in clients' sessions are utilized in team.

The core strategies in DBT are acceptance strategies, on the one hand, and behavior change strategies, on the other, with a dialectical worldview and strategies synthesizing these two poles. As noted previously, this does not mean that acceptance and change strategies are balanced equally; they are implemented as needed in any given moment. In team, their synthesis creates a stance that is ever-present: team members accept teammates just as they are, while simultaneously applying change strategies to enhance their skill and capability. DBT strategies and skills are described at length in the DBT manuals, and are only briefly reviewed here in the context of the DBT team. Once the strategies are reviewed, we will turn to several examples of how these can be put into action in Chapter 6.

While all the DBT strategies are at play in a DBT team meeting, team meetings can look very different from a DBT session in certain respects. First, team members typically come to team extremely motivated to provide effective DBT and to get help; there is typically less need to use extensive commitment strategies to get a provider to implement a change (although there are exceptions to this!). Also, DBT clinicians already know DBT. They often have already assessed their own problems and thought about at least a few strategies. The team can trust the skill of the team members, listen to what they have already sorted out and where they need help, and move forward from there. (When a team does not respect or trust a teammate, this presents a challenging problem that will be discussed in Chapter 6.) The team does not have to implement any particular strategies if they are not needed; effectiveness and doing just what works will be a useful guide for DBT teams providing therapy for the therapist.

All team members are responsible for providing therapy for the therapist. It is important for all members to remain alert, engaged, and active in providing DBT to each other. There may be times, however, when the team is uncertain about how to proceed. The observer will hopefully catch these moments; the most experienced members may also need to provide assistance to those who do not know DBT as well; and ultimately the team leader will be responsible for moving the team through any "stuck" moments.

Acceptance Strategies

The provider's motivation is one key focus of the DBT team. One of the most important factors in maintaining team members' motivation is ensuring that their team is warm, kind, compassionate, and supportive. Trust is essential. As such, a strong emphasis on acceptance strategies in team will be extremely important. When team members know that the team can provide support to offset any challenges met in the therapy room, and feel safe enough to share mistakes and uncertainties, the team can be most helpful in finding more effective ways of interacting with the client or with each other. When a team focuses only on change, team members can rapidly lose their motivation for doing this difficult work. If a teammate experiences judgment in team for the decisions made in session or elsewhere, they may stop sharing. A lack of acceptance can be problematic for the team culture, the team member, and the client. When the DBT team can provide a safe haven, a place to regroup, reenergize, and feel inspired, team members can function at their best. Even when the team feels strongly that a teammate's behavior must change, the culture of vulnerability must be maintained, through compassionate, nonjudgmental, validating responses. This safe environment creates a foundation for change strategies, as well as for a strong relationship between team members.

Validation

First and foremost, teammates will need to provide extensive validation to each other. Team members need to hear that their emotions, decisions, and challenges make sense, *even if they need to change.* All of the validation strategies discussed in DBT (Linehan, 1997) are used frequently in the DBT team. These include Level 1, listening and observing; Level 2, accurate reflection; Level 3, articulating the unverbalized; Level 4, validating in terms of sufficient causes; Level 5, validating as reasonable in the moment; and Level 6, treating the person as valid. All of these levels are essential in DBT and are just as important in the DBT team.

Level 1: Listening and Observing

This level involves paying attention. This might include making eye contact, nodding one's head while listening, and otherwise demonstrating that one is listening. This also includes noticing subtle changes in a teammate's affect or demeanor. In the DBT team, failures in Level 1 validation will most likely include things like checking one's phone during team, having side conversations, appearing to pay attention while one is actually focusing on something outside of team, or otherwise not fully attending to the speaker. One of the purposes of the observer reminder, "A team member did two things at once," is to facilitate Level 1 validation in team. This type of validation is particularly important when there is tension or conflict in the team; listening before explaining, responding, or otherwise trying to resolve the conflict will be essential in managing these situations effectively.

Level 2: Accurate Reflection

Level 2 validation involves reflecting back to a teammate their own thoughts, feelings, and overt behaviors. Doing so helps the provider feel heard and understood. Level 2 validation requires staying close to the content provided by the team member, such as summarizing what they described. This helps attain a mutual understanding of the situation and supports each team member becoming more precise and clear in describing their own reactions in and out of the therapy room.

Level 3: Articulating the Unverbalized

In Level 3, one "mind reads" unarticulated emotions and thoughts. When accurate, this level of validation is extremely powerful. The experience of having someone anticipate and understand one's reaction before it is said aloud can make one feel deeply understood. Some individuals are reluctant to use Level 3 for fear of guessing inaccurately; when this occurs, if one can simply back down (rather than insist the mind reading is correct) and collect more information, this should minimize the problems associated with inaccurate mind reading.

Level 4: Validating in Terms of Sufficient Causes

Level 4 validation communicates that a behavior (including thoughts and emotions) makes sense given its causes. These causes may include personal learning history, individual biology, or any other contextual factors. Emphasizing that every behavior has a cause, even when the behavior is undesirable or ineffective, can be invaluable in helping team members reduce judgments and understand their own behavior as well as that of teammates and clients. For example, if a team member is hesitating to directly ask a client about suicide urges due to past experience, a teammate could validate this hesitation by saying, "It makes complete sense that you are not talking about suicide directly with this client. After last month's scare with your other client, it's no wonder that you're hesitating!"

Level 5: Validating as Reasonable in the Moment

Level 5 validation involves communicating that a behavior makes sense given normative functioning and current events, or, in other words, conveying that anyone might respond in a similar way. Level 5 validation may be difficult at times in team. Validating at this level involves finding the "kernel of truth" in whatever the team member is doing, even when it is problematic, frustrating, or otherwise undesirable to the team or a client. Even if the team is focused heavily on changing a problematic behavior, it will be important to highlight how the behavior makes sense exactly as it is, and how one can understand what led the provider to engage in this behavior. For example, "I can totally understand why you are more judgmental with your client's mom. You are feeling really protective of your client, and that's a perfect storm for a lot of judgments. I think any of us might feel the same way." If one cannot find a Level 5 validation, one could move back to a Level 4 validation, stating that others might not act in this this way but that the behavior makes sense given that person's own individual history or biology. Often, however, when a team cannot validate with a Level 5, it simply means that they have not asked enough questions, or focused sufficiently on phenomenological empathy, and would benefit from pausing and deliberately searching for the kernel of truth. For example, when a teammate is expressing anger at a client in team meeting, the team can search for the ways in which this anger makes sense, and then convey this understanding to the provider, such as "I can totally see why you feel angry—I would feel the same way!"

Level 6: Treating the Person as Valid

Level 6 validation is also known as "radical genuineness." A DBT team's success relies upon team members being deeply authentic and genuine with each other. This is the opposite of treating a teammate as fragile; it assumes that a person is strong enough to be capable of hearing difficult feedback. This level also includes assuming that all team members have an inherent capability to overcome whatever difficulties they are facing in team. Being radically genuine means avoiding an overly sweet- or "fake"-sounding tone of voice, or sounding "like a therapist" instead of like a "normal person"; in other words, speaking to teammates as they might speak to their loved ones at home (with deep caring and a great deal of genuineness, and perhaps less caution). At times, speaking carefully is important, such as, "What I hear you saying is that you are feeling sad about your client"; at other times, speaking as one would to a family member can be more validating, such as, "Oh my God, I would cry my eyes out right now if that happened to my client!" Level 6 validation can also be used in seeking change; at times it is most helpful to speak carefully and say, "I am concerned we are judging our client right now," and at other times more Level 6 validation is useful: "Wow, we are being judgmental today!" Teammates will need to remain mindful of the effectiveness of their comments, and determine whether such an approach moves a particular conversation toward the goal of improved DBT.

In addition to validation, other reciprocal strategies are included as well, such as warmth, responsiveness, and collaboration. All of these acceptance strategies can be used in isolation or woven in with the other strategies discussed in this chapter. They are absolutely necessary in building the essential trust, warmth, and sense of teamwork needed to provide effective DBT.

Change Strategies

Within the context of extensive validation, DBT teams also work to improve the capability of the team member. In trying to shape each other into better DBT practitioners, using a variety of change strategies may be helpful. For some problems, validation will be sufficient, or only a brief suggestion will be needed to meet a teammate's needs. With certain problems, however, a more thorough intervention will be needed to help the provider change course with a client, enhance their skills, or regulate their emotion. The list of change strategies below is not meant to be a checklist that the team moves through exhaustively: it is merely a reminder that DBT providers have many strategies at their fingertips that they can utilize when needed. In our teams, we only infrequently need to use formal change strategies; most often brief, informal interventions are sufficient.

Problem Solving: Assessment

Assessment is an essential first step in changing any behavior. As described previously, it can be frustrating to have the team start offering solutions before understanding the problem. Oftentimes the team member will have already assessed the problem and the team can move straight to solutions; these strategies are helpful when the nature of the problem is not yet clear.

Problem Definition

First, the team and the provider must define the problem. If the team member seeking consultation cannot readily define the problem, that provider, the observer, or any other member of the team can alert the team that further definition is needed. Remember that the primary focus is on the team member's behavior, first and foremost. Client behaviors may also need to be defined. For example, if a team member was frustrated with a client, the team would identify the provider's behavior (the emotion of frustration along with any cognitions and overt behaviors that accompany the emotion), describe what it looks like (i.e., What does the team member do when frustrated?), and identify how often that the frustration is occurring, how intense it is, and how long it lasts when it occurs. The team will likely also need to define exactly what the client is doing that leads to such frustration. The team may need to ask specific questions and coach the team member to become more specific, to understand exactly what the problem is. For example, when a clinician says, "I am burned out! I am too stressed out to do this," the team might ask, "What do you mean by 'burned out'? Are you feeling frustrated? Tired? Overwhelmed? Tell us more about what you are thinking and feeling."

Problems a team might assess can occur in the therapy room, in the DBT team meeting, or elsewhere. For example:

- In the room: falling asleep in the client's presence; expressing frustration with a client in an ineffective way; not knowing how to implement a strategy with a client.
- In the DBT team meeting: arriving late; expressing judgments in team; becoming defensive when receiving feedback; not talking in team; being unwilling to provide coverage for colleagues.
- In one's personal life: *only* those behaviors that interfere with DBT treatment would be targeted by the DBT team, which might

include not sleeping well; substance abuse; problems in one's personal relationships; or working too many hours.

Behavior Analysis

Once the behavior is identified, the team can assess any relevant variables that may be useful in generating solutions. A behavior analysis examines antecedents and consequences of a particular behavior. The aim of a behavior analysis is to identify the variables controlling the behavior (i.e., which variables set off and maintain the behavior), which in turn presents opportunities for solutions. For example, the team might identify that a team member experiences anger each time clients question their competence, and the expression of that anger results in clients stopping those comments. The team may also identify that certain desired behaviors are *not* occurring; for example, the team member does not validate when the client expresses emotion, or does not assess when the client expresses higher urges for suicide. (The absence of behavior may be best addressed by a missing links analysis; see pp. 106–107.)

Chain Analysis

A chain analysis (Linehan, 1993; Linehan 2015a, 2015b) is similar to a behavior analysis, with a focus on one particular event (rather than a pattern) that includes significantly more detail. The chain analyses in team typically focus on the team member's behavior, such as the response to a client's life-threatening or therapy-interfering behavior, but the team may help the provider assess client behaviors as well. The components assessed in a chain analysis include:

- Vulnerabilities, or variables that made the individual more vulnerable to this course of events.
- The prompting event, or antecedent.
- Links between the prompting event and the target behavior, which might include thoughts, emotions, environmental events, urges, and any other intervening events.
- The team member's (or client's) identified behavior, defined as discussed above.
- Consequences, both short term and long term. Consequences are analyzed to determine if particular consequences are maintaining

a problematic behavior; often the short-term consequences reinforce the behavior, such as instant relief, and the longer-term consequences can often be utilized to deter problematic behavior, such as the shame one feels after expressing frustration with a teammate or client.

This assessment will increase understanding and highlight multiple places where solutions can be attempted. Most chains done in team are very brief, because DBT providers are already skilled at conducting chain analyses and are usually quite efficient at producing relevant information. For example, when a team member is late to team, they can do their own chain and present it to the team: "Sorry I was late. Here's my quick chain: I was sitting at my computer, and I noticed I had 5 minutes before team started. I got all excited that I could get one more session note done, but then I didn't look at my clock again until I was 5 minutes late! Somehow I lost a few minutes there. The main problem was I was just mindless and didn't keep track of time." This brief assessment can also lead right into solutions; the team member can add, "So now I know that notes take longer than 5 minutes, and I can commit to not doing that again. Also, I think I'll put an alarm in my phone so I know when I need to stand up and walk out of the room." The team can troubleshoot this commitment: "Is there anything that might get in the way of this working? How about you set that alarm right now?" Only rarely will a chain analysis in team take longer than a few minutes, such as in cases where the problem is more complicated or confusing to the team member and the team.

Missing Links Analysis

Missing links analysis (Linehan, 2015a, 2015b) is conducted when a desired behavior did not occur. It is a series of questions that attempt to identify the obstacles to behaving effectively, such as not knowing what behavior was required or needed in a particular situation, forgetting, or becoming willful. For example, if a team member agreed to use a particular intervention with a client and had not done so for several sessions, that provider could highlight this problem in team ("I seem to be avoiding bringing this topic up in session. Can you please help?") and the team could help identify the obstacles (i.e., "What got in the way?"). This analysis helps the team assess why the more effective behaviors are not occurring (e.g., the desired behavior was punished by the client or an alternative behavior was reinforced). For example, the team member may identify that they knew just what to do and did think of it in the session, but at the last second thought, "I shouldn't have to do this! My client should be able to do this on her own," which interfered with carrying out the effective strategy in session.

Many of the foregoing assessment techniques may not be needed in any given team meeting. In fact, if the team has assessed the behavior previously, understands the behavior well, but has not landed on an effective solution, most of the team time might be spent on brainstorming new solutions. Or the team member may have already identified the controlling variables and can quickly share them with the team. However, many teams tend to move to solution analysis before the problem is fully understood, so teams should take care to be sure the behavior is well defined and the controlling variables are well understood. These assessment strategies generate hypotheses to be tested. As teams identify possible controlling variables and experiment with solutions, reassessment and refinement of the plan will likely be necessary.

Problem Solving: Solution Analysis

As the important variables are identified, the team can start focusing on solutions. Solution analysis involves taking the information from the assessment and identifying one or several points where a solution could be introduced.

In terms of solutions, DBT has multiple change strategies, all of which can be effective for providers' behavior, not just clients' behaviors. These include skills, contingency management, exposure, and cognitive strategies (Linehan, 1993). Again, suggesting these strategies may not be necessary (the team member may have already implemented them, or only needs a brief reminder), but at times these specific interventions will be important.

Skills

All of the DBT skills can be implemented within the DBT team, either to alter behavior within team, as part of a plan to implement with a client, or in a team member's personal life. Referring to the skills training manuals is a standard part of the DBT team's activities and is essential for certain team problems. Team members can offer skills as solutions as often as possible. While not a comprehensive list of each specific skill, commonly used skills in team include:

1. *Mindfulness.* All of the mindfulness skills can be useful in team and in session. For example, maintaining a nonjudgmental stance with team members and clients can fundamentally change how one perceives situations and interacts with others. All team members practice one-mindfulness throughout team, and use wise mind often in team regarding themselves, teammates, and clients.

2. *Interpersonal effectiveness.* Again, all the interpersonal skills can be used in team and in therapy. DEAR MAN may be useful in requesting a teammate to change a behavior, GIVE is essential in maintaining relationships with team members, and FAST may become important if one experiences a loss of self-respect in team or believes one's point is not being heard. Identifying one's priorities prior to a difficult interaction in team can be invaluable. Finally, identifying effective levels of intensity can be useful in balancing the team culture with individual needs. (The skills of validation, dialectics, and behaviorism, also from the Interpersonal Effectiveness module, are mentioned elsewhere in this chapter.)

3. *Distress tolerance.* While the team may consider distraction, imagery, and prayer (skills from the Distress Tolerance module) during team as detracting from the team interaction, these skills may be extremely useful for team members outside of team, in and out of session. Other distress tolerance skills are highly useful in team and out: TIP, Self-Soothe, Finding Meaning, Relaxation, and other crisis survival skills can help one tolerate difficult conversations in team and with clients. The Reality Acceptance skills are invaluable in accepting each other's responses in team, clients' slow progress, and many other realities that can be difficult to tolerate. Team members' use of these skills in team will be essential in tolerating the multiple challenges involved in maintaining an effective team and treatment.

4. *Emotion regulation.* In some non-DBT clinical teams, overt expression of emotion may not be welcome, but in a DBT team where team members provide therapy to each other, the experience and expression of emotion, in a skillful, regulated manner, is highly valued. Mindfulness of Current Emotion, along with identifying emotions and understanding the model and function of emotions, can help the team identify and solve problems, as well as validate their teammate's experience. Skills

that help a clinician regulate the intensity of emotions will also be important, such as PLEASE skills and Opposite Action. Above all, maintaining a focus on emotion—for the provider and for the client—is a core part of DBT and must not be overlooked in team. Teams that regularly have meetings in which no emotions are expressed should identify this lack as a problem and actively work to increase their focus on emotion.

For example, in a DBT team, team members place themselves on the agenda, stating that they are very emotional regarding a particular client, but they don't know what the problem is. The team can suggest that the provider use the Describe skill to help the team understand the problem. This description of thoughts, sensations, and other experiences may lead the team to suggest the emotion is sadness, and further assessment could determine that the team member is sad about a painful change for the client, such as illness or the impending breakup of a romantic relationship. The team would then validate extensively, and discuss what skills might be useful for the team member, including Mindfulness of Current Emotion, Radical Acceptance, Distraction, and Problem Solving for the next therapy session.

Another example might be a team member who places themselves on the agenda to get help with intense frustration at a client's therapy-interfering behavior. The team could suggest that the provider define the client's behavior and their own reaction nonjudgmentally, then move into wise mind to determine how to move forward. In wise mind, the team member might say that they need to address the problem directly, but intense dread of the client's reaction is leading to avoidance. The team could then help their teammate to cope ahead, including scripting out what they will say, and rehearsing it either covertly or via a role play in team.

In order to successfully implement a solution, a team member may need to learn new skills (DBT skills and strategies, strategies from other evidence-based interventions, or other skills). While didactics is not the main focus of team, teaching often occurs naturally when a team is helping a teammate change a behavior. The team may teach and/or model a new therapeutic intervention or skill their teammate may use for their next session or their own personal benefit. In training teams, acquisition of new behaviors may be a significant portion of the team's intervention. For example, if a team member would benefit from using the Recovering from Invalidation skill, either for their own emotion regulation or to teach a client, the team can take the time to teach this skill either in the team meeting or at another time.

In short, the skills are just as valuable in team meetings as they are in the therapy room. DBT team members are expected to use their skills in daily life as part of providing DBT to clients; they also will benefit from using them in team meetings. These skills can be relied upon for solutions to the many types of problems team members will address in team.

Contingency Management

"Contingency management" refers to managing the consequences that occur *after* a particular behavior. Consequences can serve to increase or decrease the likelihood of that same behavior occurring in the future. The DBT team can be extremely helpful in strengthening and weakening particular team member's behaviors, both in the therapy room and in team meetings. The team manages contingencies in collaboration with the team member, through a very transparent process. These strategies are particularly useful in getting a teammate to continue to engage in difficult behaviors even when the client or other factors may work against them.

In the DBT team, the reinforcement of effective behaviors is the most commonly used contingency management strategy. A reinforcer is any consequence that increases the likelihood of a particular behavior in a similar context in the future. Reinforcement may be used to increase the likelihood of effective provider behaviors in session, in team, and at other times as well. Teams must assess what functions as a reinforcer for each teammate, and not assume it will always be praise or attention for everyone. Teammates will likely differ on what serves as a reinforcer; examples may include praise, a smile, highlighting the effectiveness of the provider's coaching or intervention, telling others about the provider's effective behavior, or letting the team member get out of the spotlight. A team discussion about which team responses function as reinforcers may be helpful.

Strengthening a desired behavior in session is an important job for the team, primarily because clients can punish effective provider behaviors, particularly if the intervention creates some distress for the client. When a team member directly discusses a difficult topic with a client, for example, a client may become distressed, shut down, appear angry, or otherwise make the team member less likely to be direct in the future. A teammate saying, "I know that was hard, but that was the most effective approach I can think of. Keep at it!" can counteract the client's reaction, and strengthen this effective therapist behavior for future sessions.

Strengthening skillful behaviors within team is also essential. A teammate may be more likely to bring up an elephant in the room, or arrive on time, or use nonjudgmental language if the team can reinforce such team-building behavior. For example, when a teammate says, "I need to talk about something but I'm embarrassed and don't want to talk about it," the other members of the team can respond, "I'm so glad you brought that up!" and provide help, which in turn can make the team member more likely to bring up additional difficult topics in the future.

The team can also be aware of effective provider behaviors outside of team and sessions. Reinforcers are highly effective in getting team members to do homework or to try new solutions in their own personal time. For example, teammates might prescribe going home and resting to address illness, or trying a DEAR MAN with a loved one to provide time to address a specific client problem or learn a new therapeutic intervention. The team member can report back to the team that they did their homework, and the team can celebrate!

Punishment, an aversive consequence that can decrease the likelihood of a behavior in the future, is also relevant to the team. Oftentimes the team is working to lessen the impact of a client punishment (as mentioned above); teammates will need to monitor for instances of effective behaviors getting punished and try to counteract the impact of clients punishing the provider. Punishment can also occur inadvertently in team; a teammate may become dysregulated when faced with a certain topic and roll their eyes, groan, or argue with another teammate, all of which might function as punishers. This has the potential to stop a team member from engaging in effective team behaviors (e.g., addressing an elephant in the room) if this behavior is not highlighted and addressed in the team meeting.

There will also be times when teammates may wish to decrease the likelihood of certain behaviors in team, such as self-invalidation in team, making judgments about a client, interrupting teammates, or reinforcing the ineffective behaviors of a client or provider. DBT team members can strategically and carefully use light forms of punishment at times, but do so with caution. Saying, "I believe you reinforced a suicidal behavior in that situation," may be an effective punisher; "You sound judgmental" and "I wish you would change how you phrased that" may also function as punishers. However, we have found that other strategies for changing behavior are much more effective in team; punishment strategies often significantly decrease a team member's motivation, and they do not teach the provider what *to* do, only what *not* to do. The punishment will also often affect the relationship of team members. Punishment may not only impact the particular behavior (e.g., self-invalidation), it may unintentionally affect others as well, such as whether a team member is willing to seek consultation more broadly, or to speak in team at all. Punishment should only be used with care, and with mindfulness of the impact of the strategy; it may be that focusing on reinforcement of an alternative behavior will be sufficient and have much less negative impact on the team member and the team. Some team members may tend to rely heavily on punishment. The team could hold a discussion to address the effectiveness of punishment and when it is helpful or harmful; the team leader or observer may be needed to help the team identify and navigate problematic behaviors in team, either with the full team or individually. A useful review of the principles of punishment can be found in Ramnerö and Törneke (2008).

A useful alternative to punishment for decreasing the frequency of a behavior is extinction, which entails eliminating reinforcers for a previously reinforced behavior. For example, the team may assess and discover that the team has reinforced a teammate judging a client by laughing or providing validation particularly when that provider is judgmental. The team can make a concerted effort to stop reinforcement for any judgmental statements, possibly combined with reinforcement for replacing the judgmental statements with validating ones.

All of these interventions can be discussed openly. Just as in DBT treatment, transparency about contingency management in the DBT team can be very useful. For example, a teammate might say in a light tone, "I am not going to reinforce that! You sounded pretty judgmental. Try restating that and then we'll go on from there."

Exposure

When a team member is avoiding a particular behavior in session or in team, particularly if the avoidance is due to anxiety, engaging in either informal or formal exposure with the team can be very helpful. For example, if one is hesitant to talk about suicide with a client out of fear of broaching that topic, the team can conduct informal exposure by bringing suicide up frequently in team, having the provider role-play bringing up suicide, and rehearsing dealing with the worst-case scenario repeatedly. Formal exposure may include developing a list of avoided topics/situations and a systematic strategy to optimize new exposure-based learning (see Craske, Treanor, Conway, Zbozinek, & Vervliet, 2014); if a team member had experienced the death of a client and was having difficulty discussing suicide even with informal exposure, the team may recommend a more extensive, formal exposure intervention.

Cognitive Strategies

Cognitive strategies may also be useful in the DBT team. Certain cognitions may interfere with effective interventions—for example, a team member engaging in judgmental thoughts may have more difficulty using acceptance strategies with a particular client. In DBT, cognitive strategies include both informal strategies, such as observing thoughts, highlighting the consequences of certain behaviors, replacing judgmental or invalidating thoughts with nonjudgmental thoughts, and increasing the frequency of validating thoughts, and formal cognitive interventions, such as Check the Facts (Linehan, 2015a, 2015b), challenging thoughts, and other common cognitive modification strategies. Ineffective thoughts will be identified during the assessment phase and can be targeted by the team with a variety of cognitive strategies.

Once solutions are generated, the team member can choose at least one solution, practice it in team if needed, then agree to implement it. Oftentimes this process is very quick, such as, "Thanks! I'll try that!" or "OK! I got what I needed! Thanks!"

Typically the more formal commitment strategies are not needed in the DBT team; DBT team members are there voluntarily and are seeking help, so they do not need their commitment strengthened. On certain occasions, however, if the provider's commitment is not strong, commitment strategies can be implemented. Pros and cons may be the most useful, for example, when discussing whether a team member will change sleep habits, meditate more often, try a wise mind exercise before a particular session, implement the behaviors role-played in the team meeting, talk more in team the following week, or simply place something on the agenda the following week. Brief rehearsal and/or troubleshooting strategies may also be helpful. These might include,

"Do you want to practice it once now, just to make sure you have it?" or "Is there anything your client might do that would throw you off your plan?" Or the team member can follow up with a teammate outside of the team meeting, such as, "Can I find one of you later to go over my plan?"

Dialectics

Just as in DBT treatment, dialectics is at the heart of the DBT team. The focus on balancing acceptance and change remains: accepting where the team member and the therapy are at while simultaneously working to change them. And once again, the balance of acceptance and change does not mean equal parts acceptance and change; instead, both poles are strongly present in each team meeting, and the emphasis on one pole or the other will depend upon what is effective for the goal of any given interaction. Maintaining a dialectical stance will involve many dialectical strategies. As summarized in Linehan (2015b), there are five major categories of dialectical strategies:

1. Overarching dialectical worldview and strategies.
2. Core strategies (problem solving vs. validation).
3. Communication-style strategies (irreverent vs. reciprocal).
4. Case management strategies (consultation to the patient vs. environmental).
5. Integrative strategies (strategies for handling specific problem situations, including suicidal behavior strategies and crisis strategies).

In the DBT team, overarching and core strategies are essential, and communication and case management strategies are implemented in specific situations. Because core and case management strategies are mentioned elsewhere in this book, only overarching and communication-style strategies will be discussed here. Integrative strategies may be referred to as an aid when helping a team member respond more effectively in session, but they are not typically used with each other in team, and therefore will not be reviewed here at all. All of these strategies are discussed in detail in Linehan (1993).

Overarching Dialectical Worldview and Strategies

Dialectical Worldview

Providing DBT therapy for the therapist requires the team to take on a dialectical worldview. One assumption of this worldview is that events are complex, with multiple components existing in a holistic relationship, with tension between polarities. This worldview suggests that opposites coexist; in other words, "truth" lies in two opposing poles rather than in one position.

A dialectical worldview facilitates synthesis when the team becomes polarized. Instead of seeking out who is "right" and who is "wrong," the team can work to incorporate the validity in both poles. This synthesis creates a whole new context from which to address the situation. For example, when a provider expresses frustration with a client's therapy-interfering behavior, instead of the team debating whether the provider should focus on phenomenological empathy and how the client's behavior makes sense, or on telling the client the behavior must stop, the team can focus on the validity in both of those poles ("It makes sense *and* it is having a negative impact on our work together"); doing so may lead to more creative, effective solutions for the situation.

Dialectics may also help when an entire team becomes polarized together, forgetting there may be another pole. Any time the team lands on a "truth," it will be essential to search for what is being left out, or the validity in the opposite pole. A team meeting is not complete without one member disagreeing or questioning the stance of the team, by saying something like, "On the other hand . . . " or "What are we leaving out?" For example, a whole team can unite in frustration against an external, non-DBT provider, or an administrator, without pausing to see that person's perspective. The observer and all members can watch for consensus in the team, which may be a warning sign that the team is polarized and not including both poles in the discussion or situation. Clinical decision making is improved by attending to multiple perspectives and nonjudgmental disagreement in the team.

This worldview leads team members to see situations as transactional, meaning that there is no single cause to any situation or behavior. Instead, two poles influence each other continuously over time. In other words, a provider's behavior influences the client, which reciprocally influences the provider in return, repeatedly, in an ongoing transaction. For example, assuming a client caused difficulty in a therapeutic relationship, without also seeing one's own contribution, would be nondialectical; it is important for team members to identify both client and provider contributions over time, throughout multiple interactions, when discussing this type of problem in team. The same principle applies to situations where a team member blames a parent or other provider; to be dialectical, the team would search for transactional influence from all those involved.

Dialectical Strategies

In addition to a dialectical worldview, the same dialectical strategies used in DBT treatment (Sayrs & Linehan, 2019; Linehan, 1993) can be implemented in the DBT team. While all of the dialectical strategies are relevant in team, the ones most commonly relied upon are as follows:

1. *And* versus *but*. The language used by team members can be made more dialectical by emphasizing the word *and* instead of the word *but*. For example, when a provider struggles with, "I really like my client, *but* I can't tolerate this particular behavior," this suggests the two statements are at odds with each other and cannot coexist. When the team moves the language to "I like my client *and* I can't tolerate her behavior," the statement acknowledges both poles are true at once; the team is no longer pressured to decide whether the team member continues working with the client, and instead starts seeking ways to continue working with the client *and* address the problem that is stretching the team member's limits, or care about the client deeply *and* move toward therapy vacation or termination.

2. *Making lemonade out of lemons.* This dialectical strategy is very similar to the DBT skill of Finding Meaning (Linehan, 2015a, 2015b), in which the team helps the team member find the opportunity or value in a difficult situation. It is important to emphasize the dialectical nature of this strategy: rather than moving from distress to seeing only the "good" in a situation (moving from one pole to the other), one can see the pain *and* the benefit. For example, the nondialectical statement, "My client expressed a lot of frustration with me, but it's a 'good' thing because I am learning from it," would instead be stated as, "My client expressed frustration with me. I hated it! At the same time, I can see that I will learn a lot from this situation."

3. *Stories and metaphors.* Just as clients can at times have difficulty seeing the other pole, a team member may also struggle. In such

a situation, using a metaphor or story can facilitate more openness to seeing both sides of a situation. For example, when one might be hesitant to conduct exposure with a client, the team might liken the situation to walking across hot coals to reach a loved one, a difficult journey with a highly desired result. Telling a team member they need to do exposure might be met with more fear; using a metaphor, analogy, or personal story can broaden one's perspective and therefore increase dialectical thinking and willingness.

Communication-Style Strategies

A balance of style is important within a DBT team, as well: balancing reciprocity with irreverence can be important to maintaining movement, speed, and flow in the team. Using heightened drama, unorthodox responses, and especially humor, in juxtaposition with warmth and validation, will keep the team discussion flowing. For example, when most members of the team are warmly validating a provider's fear at a client's recent suicide attempt, having one teammate exclaim "Holy s*&t!" can break the mood and keep the team from getting stuck.

Each teammate will likely tend toward one style or the other; however, as in DBT itself, all team members must be able to implement both reciprocal and irreverent styles. As discussed elsewhere, some shaping may be needed to tolerate irreverence in team. Irreverence is not sarcasm and is not mean-spirited: instead, it is a nonjudgmental, novel response used to grab attention. Team members will need to discriminate between irreverence and sarcasm and discuss judgments when they occur, as well as any defensiveness. The team can talk about judgments openly when this occurs; it will be important to give feedback in these situations.

It could be easy for any team member to become overwhelmed at the number of strategies listed here. In reality, therapy for the therapist will likely not look like a set of strategies, it will look like a warm, supportive, helpful discussion among teammates. In most teams, these discussions are brief as well, due to time limitations. Oftentimes providers have already thought through much of the problem, and may need very specific, brief help to be able to move forward. It will be important for teams to remain effective, do what works, and not get slowed down by trying to use every strategy. Most of the time, therapy for the therapist is straight-forward and brief. If the team's interventions are not helpful, the discussion can be returned to in the next team meeting.

To illustrate the brevity of a team's intervention, we've included the following example:

PROVIDER: Team, I could use some help! I'm super frustrated with my client. I got really mad yesterday in session. I'm requesting help with assessment, because clearly I'm missing something. I think some validation will help bring my anger down too.

TEAMMATE: Do you know what set it off?

PROVIDER: It was when my client told me she had left her diary card at home. Normally I wouldn't be so upset, but we talked about this problem in last session, and I even texted her during the week. Somehow, she still forgot it. I tried to assess in session, but that's where I'm stuck. I can't figure out why this keeps happening despite all my work.

TEAMMATE: First, that sounds totally frustrating! I would be mad too. Second, tell us what you know already about this diary card, then we can add a few more ideas.

[The provider describes when the client typically does her diary card, that she always brought it in before, but then suddenly stopped.]

TEAMMATE: Seems like something changed, if she was pretty regular about the card before. It'd be helpful if you could assess when the change occurred. Did her daily routine change? Or did something happen when you reviewed her card with her right before that?

PROVIDER: Of course! It stopped right after she told me she was really embarrassed about putting something on her diary card. I forgot all about that. She got frustrated with me in that session because I didn't realize how much shame she had about it. I'll try to assess more about that session, and see if there's some shame or anger at me. Thanks so much—that is all I need for now, I'll check in again next week if I still feel stuck.

Therapy for the Therapist May Be Insufficient

As discussed previously, the team must remain vigilant for team member problems that are too extensive or intense for the team to handle. While the team does provide therapy for the therapist, the role of the DBT team member does *not* include becoming a provider for teammates. Team members are fellow professionals and colleagues and should avoid becoming medication managers, individual therapists, or mediators for each other. If significant meeting time is spent on the same problem repeatedly, or the problem does not seem to be changing sufficiently, or the team simply does not have the time or expertise to manage the problem, the team may recommend that a particular team member receive professional help outside of team. This might be in the form of trauma treatment, sleep intervention, couples therapy, or many other interventions.

Many problems will simply be accepted, or will require minimal intervention using strategies in this chapter. But for problems that are more challenging, that have not responded to the team's attempts at solutions, and are not tolerable, other measures may be necessary. Teams should not continue interventions that are not working, and should not attempt to solve problems outside of their area of competence. If the roles become confusing or certain members are uncomfortable with the level or type of intervention, this kind of problem should be discussed in team and alternate solutions considered. When team problems do not respond to the strategies in this chapter, an outside consultation may be helpful. This could be from a DBT expert, an administrator, or anyone with a fresh perspective and skill in managing interpersonal conflict.

There may also be situations that are creating problems in team or with clients in which the provider is not willing to discuss the problem in team. To maintain the collegial, caring, voluntary tone in team, these issues should not be forced out into the open in a DBT team. The team leader will be essential in such a case. The team leader might review team agreements and try to build motivation one-on-one and/or help this individual prepare something for team discussion. The team leader may also help this individual obtain resources outside of team, if relevant. Forcing issues out of a reluctant teammate will not only upset that team member, but it may make all members hide vulnerabilities.

Conclusion

Therapy for the therapist is truly the backbone of the DBT team. This starts with a foundation of validation; therapy for the therapist will only work if each team member feels safe enough to be vulnerable and open in team. Trust, compassion, and care are essential. Within this context of warmth and acceptance, team members can place themselves on the agenda, highlight which obstacles are interfering with effective treatment, and request help. These obstacles can include emotion, problematic contingencies, lack of skill or knowledge, or many other issues. The team can then use the above strategies to help the clinician move the treatment forward for one or several clients, by way of treating the team member. It is important to remember that there are no set rules or protocols for helping team members; these interventions may take 30 seconds and the provider is able to move forward again, or they may be more formal and occur across several team meetings. Each team member will need to remain alert for what is needed, using DBT principles and strategies.

IDEAS FOR PRACTICE

- Practice using all six levels of validation in one team meeting.
- Notice your first reaction when a teammate describes a mistake. Experiment with validating them first, before offering solutions. Ask your teammate for feedback.
- Practice defining behaviors in team. All team members identify a target behavior they are trying to change, and the team can practice making those descriptions more precise.
- Practice chain analyses on each other. Use a whiteboard or projector so that the entire team can see the chain. Try to identify the controlling variables (i.e., the variables that seem most influential over the behavior).
- Practice missing links analysis with a teammate who committed to a particular behavior and did not follow through.
- Practice listing as many solutions for a team member's chain as possible.
- For a particular problem, choose one solution and have every member of the team rehearse it in front of the rest of the team.
- Discuss which team behaviors function as reinforcers for each member, and which function as punishers.
  - Team members write about a situation in which the team's response increased their willingness to have hard conversations. What did the team do? Why did it work?
  - Then members write about a team's response that decreased their willingness to engage in difficult tasks for the benefit of the team. Why didn't those work?

- • Team members share with the team what they wrote, using a nonjudgmental stance and the Describe skill.
- • Discuss and summarize for the entire team.

▨ Have a team discussion about the use of punishment in team. When is it helpful? When is it harmful?

▨ Practice saying something direct to a teammate. Start with low-intensity comments, such as, "I don't really like your shirt," even if that is not true. Have every team member say something like this to someone in team. Discuss the challenges in being direct with each other. Gradually work up to direct feedback about a client or an event in team, using the Describe skill. Be sure to balance such direct comments with warmth and validation. Practice reinforcing direct communication with each other.

▨ Practice irreverent lines. Practice giving one reciprocal and one irreverent line for the same situation. Share with teammates.

▨ Have a team discussion about when irreverence can turn sarcastic, judgmental, or mean-spirited, and how you want to handle that as a team.

▨ Ask a teammate to conduct exposure with you for a behavior that you have been avoiding.

▨ Label strategies used with other members of the team each time you notice them.

CHAPTER 6

Responding to Problems in the DBT Team

I t is expected that teams will have problems on a regular basis. In fact, if a team has no tension or difficult moments, it is likely not being dialectical! Because problems are inevitable, teams will need a way to identify and address them. As we talked about in Chapter 5, many of the same DBT principles that are useful in therapy will apply to addressing team problems.

Most problems will be quickly solved, with a brief comment or intervention such as feedback from the observer, an irreverent comment, or a simple request to change something. Typically, team problems will not need extended time to resolve them. And many problems will not need a solution at all! In fact, team members may experience fatigue if they attempt to process every problem. When discussing which problems to address, it will be extremely important to remain mindful of the goal, which is to provide DBT with fidelity, making sure team members have sufficient skill and capability to keep the team and treatment moving forward. The key to dealing with team problems is to know which problems to ignore and which to target, based on which problems actually interfere with this goal. While focusing on change, teammates can simultaneously radically accept the state of the team, behaviors of other team members, the struggles of each individual member, the pace of progress, and those problems that are not solvable in that moment, exactly as acceptance is used by DBT providers with their own clients. All team members will need to accept something they do not like, at least some of the time!

This chapter focuses on addressing those problems that pose obstacles to fidelity to DBT in teams. Additionally, for teams that are running well, these strategies may also be useful in monitoring the health of the team, fine-tuning, preventing problems, and enjoying successes in team.

Prevention

Preventing team problems before they start is ideal. One major purpose of the agenda, roles, and other structure discussed in this book is to help keep the team on track and prevent problems. Of course, not all problems can be prevented, and, in fact, waiting for certain problems to arise before introducing a lot of structure can be a useful strategy. Even so, we recommend certain strategies to help prevent problems, including:

1. Have an orienting and commitment conversation with each member as they join the team, and again as necessary. Doing so will make sure that everyone on the team agrees to certain structure and practices. This gives each member of the team permission to call out and address problems as they arise, without fear that certain individuals have a different understanding of how the team is run and what the team's goals are.

2. Follow the DBT team agreements. The agreements provide the structure and practices to help team members mindfully attend to what happens in team, avoid problems in team, and wrestle with them when they do arise. This includes maintaining a nonjudgmental stance with each other, providing therapy for the therapist, and focusing on offering highly effective treatment with fidelity. The agreements also help create a safe place to challenge each other, explore what is being left out, and talk about what causes distress.

3. Balance structure with flexibility. On the one hand, becoming rigid with the agreements and team structure will likely hurt the team, rather than help it. On the other hand, changing the structure because a teammate is distressed may lead to avoidance, reinforcement of problematic behaviors, and other problems. Thoughtfully creating and agreeing to the structure and sticking to it is important. As the team evolves, mindful discussions of which components may need to change can help the team adapt the structure in a strategic, careful way.

4. Validate each other and maintain phenomenological empathy for every member of the team.

5. Develop a culture wherein the behaviors that are effective for the team get reinforced by all members (not just the leader).

6. Emphasize what is going well—in team, with clients, and for individual team members. Most teams have multiple strengths; if problems are the only focus, the team can lose sight of the effective strategies already developed. When problems are seen within a context of successes, they take on less power than if they are the sole focus of the team.

7. Check in with each other. Schedule annual retreats, or set aside occasional team time to ask how the team is doing. Such conversations can become a part of the team routine. Create a platform for team members to give input, shape the team, and contribute to its culture.

8. Spend time together outside of team. Maintaining the health of the team requires a fair amount of trust in each other, which will not happen without time to interact and get to know each other. Engaging in occasional social activities together and sharing some amount of personal information will help build the camaraderie and trust that can facilitate vulnerability in team.

9. Have fun! Develop a team culture of humor and silliness to balance the at times very serious topics addressed in team.

10. Accept the team. This chapter focuses heavily on change and developing solutions. To maintain the central dialectic in DBT, this focus on change must be balanced with a strong emphasis on acceptance. All teams will have tension, it is a necessary component of any team committed to a dialectical stance. All teams will experience moments of frustration between members. Some team meetings will feel unhelpful. It is important to deeply accept the idea that the team will never be perfect. This acceptance also includes individual team members who may frustrate, worry, or annoy others. Every team member will have a "quirk," an "Achilles' heel," or behaviors that are at times problematic. These individual differences are necessary for teams to experience thesis, antithesis, and synthesis. Not every quirk or difference must be discussed until it is "solved." Allowing some problems to lie is as important as the strategies provided here. Other problems may take time to solve, or take lower priority as other, more urgent problems are addressed. Teams can evaluate whether solving the problem is necessary, or whether it is more effective to "love the quirk," wait it out, or all of the above.

Identifying Problems

Sometimes team problems are glaringly obvious, but often there is a subtle elephant in the room that is difficult to pinpoint. Frequently, the team leader, observer, or the team as a whole will notice a shift in the team interaction. This may happen gradually, or the change may be abrupt due to events such as a new member joining, a client's suicide, or any other event that changes the team's culture.

First, simple observation can highlight team problems. It is every teammate's responsibility to identify problems in the team culture, including members becoming gradually more judgmental, or members not addressing issues with each other's implementation of DBT. Team will not run effectively if team members notice a problem and wait for the team leader or observer to become aware of and solve it. All team members must skillfully express their own distress and call out elephants in the room. Such problems can be broached in the team, or one can first seek guidance from the team leader privately. The topic can then go on the agenda for a team discussion if needed.

We have also used scheduled team check-ins to identify problems, even when the team seems to be running smoothly. This can help catch issues early, and team members often appreciate knowing there is a regular system for discussing their concerns. Such a check-in can be done in team, at a retreat, or one-on-one. Doing so once a year can be sufficient when there are no obvious problems (this serves to prevent problems); greater frequency may be needed for certain periods of time, when, for whatever reason, more attention to team functioning may be necessary.

It is helpful to add structure to a check-in by assigning a question or a topic to prompt the conversation. Reserve a fair amount of time for these conversations (e.g., 30 minutes), or plan to return to them over multiple meetings. When giving a prompt, we find it most useful to give the team a moment to reflect and prepare, then have each member address the prompt in turn, with no response from others until everyone has had their turn. We have also found that first doing a "free-write" can be useful: each member writes for several minutes in response to a prompt, then each member shares their response in turn. This approach seems to minimize members being influenced by others and changing their answers, and may result in better information for the team.

Prompts for these check-ins should be tailored to your own situation. Some prompts we have used in our teams include:

- What are two things you do in team that are effective for the team? What are two things you do that are ineffective?

- What are the top two elements of our team that work well for you? And what are the top two things you would like to change?

- Review the team agreements. Where does the team adhere to the agreements, and where has it drifted? Do you have hesitation or concern related to any of the agreements?

- Where are your limits stretched? What habits have you developed that may be difficult to maintain over the long term? Are there things the team does or requests of you that stretch your limits?

- Reflect on a situation when the team increased your willingness to have hard conversations. What did team do? Why did it work? And what has the team done that decreased your willingness to engage in difficult tasks for the benefit of the team? Why didn't those work?

- How do you handle feeling criticized or embarrassed? How might the team know you are feeling this way? Do you like how you handle these situations? If not, how might you make that response effective for yourself, your team, and your clients?

- What types of influence do you have? How does it affect your behavior on team? Is it effective? What other types of influence do you see in the team? Everyone in a team has different types of power or influence over other members and over the team culture overall. Some team members have a lot of power because of their role within the agency or group (e.g., they are the boss or supervisor to some or all of the team members). Others might have a different type of influence because of extensive experience, training, or expertise. Others may have significant influence because they are adored or viewed as fragile, and no one wants to hurt their feelings, or because they have a strong aversive reaction to certain statements in team. For example, if one individual becomes extremely defensive every time the conversation turns toward in-team behaviors, that individual may have a significant influence over the team discussion.

Team members may have strong urges to just dive in and break a topic wide open in team, with a more confrontational or blunt style. Often this is the most helpful and efficient way to go; however, with team members who are not yet desensitized to very direct communication, the team may need to do some coaching and easing in. And some teams just prefer a softer touch. This is OK! Remember the goal is to help the team become more effective; it will be important to mindfully choose ways to proceed that move the whole team toward the goal.

Urges to avoid may be strong for some problems. While it can be effective to ignore issues that are not interfering with team goals, the team will need to address problems that disrupt team functioning. Avoidance prevents solution generation, and also communicates that some topics are taboo or too difficult. If tensions are high in the team, and there is reluctance to discuss these topics openly, the team leader may conduct 1:1 or 1:2 meetings with team members. It should be made very clear that the team leader is not responsible for solving all of these problems, but is merely facilitating assessment, consolidating information, and guiding the team toward dealing with the problems. The responsibility for solving problems remains with the team, not with any one individual; otherwise the solutions may not feel satisfying or useful. Information gained in 1:1 meetings will typically come back to the whole team (assuming it is relevant to the whole team) for discussion.

For example, during a particularly stressful time in my (JS) team, we attempted to identify the problem in team and found we were unable to. In my role as team leader, I realized more information was needed. I decided to meet with each member of the team, either individually or in small groups, to try to figure it out. I asked every member the same questions, which were fairly generic because I wanted to cast a wide net to identify the problems:

- "Is there anything you would like to see changed in our team practice?"
- "How do you feel about the role of the team leader? Is it working for you?"
- "Would a retreat be helpful to you? And would that consist of just social time or also exercises/ways to build the team?"
- "How do you feel about the team size?"
- "What is working well in team?"
- "Do you want to comment on anything else?"

These questions led to identifying that the size of the team seemed to be the heart of the problem; team members felt they did not have enough time to get their needs met, and felt distanced from others in the team (at that time, our team was quite large). I also received other interesting information, including that there was some frustration with me as team leader regarding team size, and that some did not understand that they could bring a problem forward themselves, and were waiting for me to identify and solve the problem. Overall, I was able to focus in on the main problem, and also reset some team expectations in these meetings, then lead the team in a discussion about team size. After a few discussions of the pros and cons, we ended up breaking the team into two separate teams.

During this period, I also graphed the team's satisfaction at each team meeting, as measured by ratings of overall satisfaction and on several specific items (e.g., satisfaction with size of team, irreverence in team, and amount of help received in team). I displayed these graphs in team on a regular basis. This conveyed an openness to feedback and desire to address problems in the team, which seemed to go a long way toward improving team morale in a trying time. While fairly simplistic, these types of data can facilitate communication in team, define problems, and get everyone motivated to start solving problems.

This is not to say that every team will need to take heroic measures to address a team problem. Typically, team problems are resolved quickly when the team focuses directly on them. The above example was a particularly difficult team problem, and the problem itself (team size) inhibited the team's ability to resolve it in a team meeting. We have had to resort to this type of intensive intervention only once in a long history with this team.

Not all informal assessment needs to happen face to face. Asking individuals to turn in written answers or conducting surveys online can work as well. This may give team members the opportunity to respond anonymously, which at certain points may be necessary. When communication and trust in a team is damaged, anonymous assessment may be an excellent starting point for improving communication, by giving the team leader some ideas of where to focus attention. The team leader can then support the team in moving to discussions in person, based on this information.

Formal assessment measures are another useful way of identifying where problems lie and beginning a dialogue. These measures can also be readministered and used to monitor change over time. Below are just a few examples of instruments teams may use; measures may be chosen based on the particular issues and needs of a team. These measures can be given to each team member in or outside of team, then discussed as a group. The team leader can consolidate the answers and provide talking points to the group.

- Copenhagen Burnout Inventory (Kristensen, Borritz, Villadsen, & Christensen, 2005), a measure of burnout in human services fields that assesses personal, work-related, and client-related distress.
- Maslach Burnout Inventory (Maslach & Jackson, 1981), a commonly used measure of burnout in human services fields that assesses depersonalization, emotional exhaustion, and personal accomplishment.
- Barriers to Implementation (Chugani, Mitchell, Botanov, & Linehan, 2017), a measure of barriers to DBT implementation including team, administrative, philosophical/theoretical, and structural problems.

Assessing what is going well is just as essential as assessing problems. Without such assessment, the team leader and members, as well as the team at large, can become quite demoralized if bombarded with lists of problems. Also, if the team is not very mindful of the effective components of the team, necessary resources won't be focused on maintaining those useful elements. This can be accomplished by simply asking what team members like about the team, which components they do not want to change, and what is working well for them.

Placing the Problem on the Agenda

When a problem is broached by a team member, whether it is the team leader, observer, or another member of the team, that provider is placed on the agenda. The topic is then addressed in a direct, descriptive, concrete, dialectical manner. This means focusing on describing the behavior or problem to the team, placing the main focus on oneself and one's own reaction to the problem. For example, "I've noticed we had a lot of judgments in team today, and we didn't highlight and restate all of them. I see why this happened—talking about that particular client made several of us, including me, really frustrated! I'm worried we might be drifting from our agreements, and that this might affect our feedback and decisions today." If the team in return can communicate that the problem description made sense and had validity to it in some regard, this will facilitate the discussion and reinforce the behavior of highlighting the problem.

Defining the Problem Behaviorally

Once someone has identified a problem to the team, the team can decide if further definition is needed. This may begin with a simple conversation in team. Many of the problems identified will relate to an individual team member's behavior, and the strategies discussed in Chapter 5 (Therapy for the Therapist) for defining behavior can be used. At other times, however, the problem will be more team-based, where the culture of the team has drifted away from the agreements. For example, an entire team stops putting the team member on the agenda, and reverts back to focusing solely on clients' problems, or the team gradually becomes less behavioral and specific in its language.

Regardless of whether the problem involves one member or multiple members of a team, the process of defining the behavior is the same as in individual DBT. The definition should include a topographical description of observable behavior, with no added concepts, assumptions, interpretations, or judgments. For example, a team might describe one particular member as "invalidating." While it is important to identify problematic interactions in team, this single word does not actually state what the individual said or did. A better definition of the behavior might be: "On Tuesday in team, you said, 'You shouldn't feel so sad about your client.' That felt invalidating, as though my emotions were not valid. This has happened on other occasions as well." The behavior is defined by a specific example and an actual quote, which will help each team member fully understand which behaviors are being addressed.

Another example is telling a team member they "do not care" about team. This definition is not concrete or specific, and also assumes a great deal about what the individual is thinking and intending. A clearer definition might be, "You have arrived late for 3 weeks in a row, and when you are here you check your phone several times. Can you tell us what is going on?" If a member does not define the behavior sufficiently, the team can ask a member to restate certain items in order to become more specific. For example, if a person states, "The team is harsh sometimes," the team will need to know exactly what "harsh" means. And again, not every problematic behavior must be discussed; problems will be brought up if and when they are creating problems for the team and/or a specific member.

Problem Solving

The team does not have to spend a lot of time defining; the definition does not need to be perfect, it just needs to be sufficient to help the team move on to solutions. Once the team has a reasonable definition and understanding of the problem, problem solving can begin. Chapter 5 gave an overview of ways in which DBT strategies can be used to generate team solutions. Before reviewing examples, we will briefly review some overarching principles that can guide every team member in the course of problem-solving team difficulties.

1. Take a stance that is flexible, not rigid. We have returned to this mantra multiple times throughout this book. Instead of focusing on rules or a single "right" way to proceed, use principles to guide decisions. Focus on the team's agreements, goals, and DBT strategies to identify the best path forward for the team.

2. Remain nonjudgmental; use the Describe skill and behavioral definitions. Doing so will provide the team with the clearest possible information, help everyone stick to the facts, and keep emotion at a less-intense level. Once judgments and vague language become predominant, the team can lose valuable information as well as the motivation to move forward.

3. Speak up when there is a problem. If there are concerns about bringing the topic up with the entire team, having a conversation with the team leader or another team member may be a useful first step, particularly when there are barriers to a full-team discussion.

4. Attend to team members' emotion. The majority of team problems seem to involve team members becoming frustrated, sad, ashamed, fearful, angry, and so on. Often a provider's emotion is the core to the difficulty in team. Fortunately, this is a team of DBT clinicians who know

just what to do with emotion! Identifying and working with the emotion in team will be essential to solving just about any team problem. The principles of emotion regulation, along with the use of skills worksheets as needed, can help label and navigate emotion in team. Remember: emotions serve a function, and can convey important information to the team member and the team. The team can validate, help the provider address vulnerabilities, decide whether to use problem solving and/or opposite action, and incorporate any other relevant skills. (See Linehan, 2015a, 2015b, for a detailed description of emotion regulation skills.)

5. Validate each other. Listen to the problem first, before responding. Remember that for any behavior that is frustrating, baffling, or in any other way problematic, there is an explanation that makes sense. All behavior is caused. Find the kernel of truth, and communicate how the provider's and the client's emotions, thoughts, urges, and overt behaviors make sense. Use the GIVE skill with each other. Remember that members of the team are likely already trying very hard to follow the agreements and be helpful to their teammates. A healthy dose of validation, support, and sense of *team* is invaluable in doing this very difficult work.

6. Remain dialectical. Balance acceptance and change effectively. The team will need to find the validity in the problematic behavior or situation, *and* be straightforward about the problems it is causing. Attending to and validating both poles will be most likely to lead to synthesis. For example, when a teammate appears annoyed with the team's suggestion, while the team will likely give feedback about the annoyance, the team can also note that the annoyance was caused. Although annoyance may not have been communicated effectively, there is some kernel of truth to be found, which might include something that the team did not assess fully. Finding and validating the kernel of truth on both poles can help with motivation and problem solving. Being dialectical in style will also help. Irreverence is extremely useful to help a team or provider when they are stuck, but being only irreverent is a problem. Similarly, being warm is very important, but being only warm can also lead to difficulties.

7. Address willfulness in team. "Willfulness" refers to a moment when a teammate fights reality, tries to control, gives up, or otherwise does not do just what is needed in the moment. Simply highlighting can help: in a light voice, asking, "Are you feeling willful?," can bring awareness to the moment. The team can also help explore what the threat

might be (willfulness often comes from some type of threat; see Linehan, 2015a, 2015b), such as losing something important or experiencing a negative outcome. For example, when a team member's limits are stretched too far, they may feel their peace of mind and free time are threatened, and become willful around providing necessary extra time to a particular client; or a team member may feel a team suggestion is a threat to their relationship with their client (such as saying no to a client, or recommending the client start exposure or another therapeutic intervention the client will not like). Helping the team member identify and grapple with that threat can also help loosen willfulness. Ultimately, acceptance will be needed for moments of willfulness; trying to force willfulness to stop is simply more willfulness. If the team can remain curious and open, eventually the willfulness will pass. Again, teammates can use skills handouts and worksheets as needed to assess and address willfulness.

8. Assess carefully. Using all the DBT assessment tools will help the team understand the problem. (At the same time, do not get stuck assessing so long that there are no solutions!)

9. Offer solutions, and don't give up when they do not seem helpful. Keep assessing and brainstorming until there is some movement. Consider all relevant DBT change strategies: skills, exposure, contingency management, and cognitive strategies.

10. At the same time, not everything must be solved. Each member of the team will need Radical Acceptance, Half-Smile, Willing Hands, and a lot of mindfulness to tolerate the many problems with clients and teammates that simply will not get solved. Some problems will not rise to the top of the priority list, or will take much longer to solve than team members wish. Team members may decide to "love the dandelions" (Linehan, 1993) and turn their attention elsewhere.

11. Once the solutions are identified, the team can check to be sure that there is a commitment to implementing the solution, and address any potential obstacles, if needed.

Common Problems Arising in DBT Teams

We have included a rather long list of example problems that may occur in any DBT team. This is not to say that all teams are headed toward all of these problems; rather than pare down the list of examples, we included many, in the hopes it will normalize any problems that arise and provide some direction for how to address them. We divided these problems into two categories: problems occurring with one member of the team, and problems occurring with the team at large. Of course, there can be overlap between individual and team problems. While it may oversimplify problems somewhat, we organized them in this way for the sake of clarity. The solutions offered here are just a few examples of what teams might do to address such problems; they are merely suggestions, not a prescribed list of interventions. Each team should take care to assess carefully and use solutions that closely fit their own unique problem.

Problems That Occur with One Team Member

Treatment Is Stuck

One of the main tasks in DBT team is to help improve client outcomes. The most common team problem we have encountered is when a team member is chronically stuck with a client and repeatedly returns to the team with the same problem and little movement, and team suggestions have not improved the outcome. This may be due to not implementing the solutions suggested, or not having a clear conceptualization, or responding to the "crisis of the week," where therapy targets shift each week based on the most urgent or pressing matter, such that no strategic plan or change can be maintained. Often, when treatment is not moving forward and the team is not helpful, the problem is assessment: the team is not fully understanding the problem, and therefore the solutions are not aimed at the right problem. One of the least effective responses from a team is throwing multiple solutions at the team member without fully understanding the problem; remembering the team agreement to assess before solving is essential in this case. The team can simply ask a lot of questions, and/or review the case formulation, to see how the provider is organizing the treatment. Inevitably, the team has more insight and better suggestions once they've seen the problem (as opposed to just talking about it), so watching a video of one or more sessions or demonstrating the problem through role plays may be helpful. These assessment strategies can help lead to an intervention such as problem solving (brainstorming then evaluating and trying out solutions). The team can also help their teammate accept the slow pace of progress, and, perhaps, help to evaluate whether DBT is right for this client.

A Teammate Repeatedly Says, "I've Already Tried That!"

We have seen many teams struggle with one provider in the team who repeatedly responds with "I've already tried that!" or "That won't work!" to just about every solution suggested in team. This may come across at times as hopeless, irritable, or defensive. There is a dialectic here: if the team does not understand the problem thoroughly, the team member may be accurate in saying that all of the solutions provided are insufficient. It may be that further assessment will help resolve the problem. At the same time, the provider may be missing something important in the team's feedback. They may not have tried the solutions offered, or have done them less comprehensively than the team suggested, or may not even know how to implement a particular solution. When a team member refuses most suggestions, a first intervention could be to figure out what was *actually* tried in session, not just a description of what happened. Once again, watching video, conducting role plays, and other careful assessment may be needed to uncover why the solutions haven't worked. This is done in a collegial, "We are all figuring this out together" style. Second, if a team member is defensive or willful during these discussions, once again assessing "What's the threat?" may also be useful. As described previously in this chapter, this involves highlighting the defensive reaction, and assessing what might feel threatening about this conversation. For example, a teammate might say, "I worry I've made you feel defensive. Is that true? What sparked that response?" The team member might feel that their reputation or credibility, or their sense of progress with a client, is threatened. Assessing emotions and thoughts pertaining to their reactions may help open the conversation such that more solutions become available. Importantly, a team member who turns down every solution often ends up punishing the team's help, which can lead everyone toward giving up. A third intervention might be for the observer, team leader, or another team member to highlight this problem by saying, "I notice you're turning down all of our solutions. Can we talk about that? I am worried we are going to give up."

There may come a time when the team simply disagrees with a therapist's approach or formulation. In this case, all members of the team will need to listen nonjudgmentally to each other and acknowledge the disagreement. In high-risk situations, the team may want to be more directive (e.g., if they believe the therapist is not taking the client's suicide risk seriously enough, they may say, "Listen, this is life and death, and we're really concerned about your client right now"), and if that is not sufficient, the team leader may need to intervene. For other problems, running experiments (e.g., the team can say to the therapist, "Try it that way in the next session, and if it doesn't work, will you try what we are suggesting?"), highlighting that the team is not in agreement, and even simply letting another week pass can help. While the team does not give mandates, it will be important for the therapist to be open to feedback and acknowledge the team has expressed concern about the approach.

A Teammate Is Judgmental

Another common problem we have seen is judgments in team. At times, this can become a problem for an entire team as it slowly and steadily drifts from the agreements; at other times it is one individual who relies on judgmental explanations and descriptions, which impacts the tone of the entire team. Hopefully, the provider will have already agreed to a nonjudgmental stance when joining the team, so the primary intervention is often to briefly highlight the judgment (e.g., "There was some judgment in there!" or "Is that a judgment?"). The observer can also note judgments as they arise, by ringing the bell or otherwise bringing the team's attention to them, then using the Describe skill or other relevant skills. In many of these cases, reviewing the rationale for a nonjudgmental stance (e.g., sticking to the facts leads to more effective solutions and keeps emotions more regulated) is sufficient.

If the judgments persist, another intervention may be to assess the function of the behavior. We worked with one individual who identified, through assessment in team, that the judgments he made helped him to feel validated by the team, and describing the client without judgments left him feeling the team did not fully understand the intensity and difficulty of the situation. In such a case, the team can help by providing more intense validation for descriptions, and less validation when judgments were used (contingency management). This type of approach should be discussed openly, with the team member fully involved in the development of such a plan. In another case, a team member identified intense fear of a client's high suicide risk, and the judgments functioned to suppress the fear. A team in this situation might respond by blocking the avoidance, validating the difficulty of the emotion, helping problem-solve to reduce the risk, and supporting acceptance of the uncertainty of working with suicidal clients.

Not all judgments are worth halting the team conversation to address. Judgments are a common part of our culture's language and occur frequently. The observer and all teammates can determine if the judgment is affecting the team meeting, a team member, or a client, or if it can be ignored. Teams may at times choose to ignore judgments until a pattern emerges that the team determines needs to be addressed.

A Teammate Defines Problems in Vague Terms

A team member may use nonjudgmental language when describing a problem, but the definition is too vague for the team to provide help. This can lead the team to provide ineffective solutions, or invalidate the team member, because the problem is not well understood. The solution to this problem can be to ask the provider to offer a more specific definition; for example, if a team member asks for help dealing with a client who is "defensive," the team can respond, "Can you be more specific?" or "What are the actual behaviors you are talking about?" In general, the definition needs to be specific enough that everyone in team has the same understanding of the problem. A more precise definition may also be needed if a provider describes a diagnosis instead of a behavior. For example, when a team member says, "My client is anxious," the team may have multiple interpretations of what this term means; the team can ask for more specificity, and the provider can clarify, "She is having panic attacks that last a few minutes each morning before leaving for school."

We have seen teams get bogged down in trying to define behaviors. The team should only spend enough time on this topic to obtain an effective, usable definition of the behavior. It does not need to be more detailed than is needed to help the team member. The team can then add more detail as needed, as problem solving progresses.

A Teammate Is Invalidating

Many teams have struggled with a team member who frequently makes comments that are experienced as invalidating by other members. Invalidation can take a variety of forms: telling teammates how they "should" feel, or telling others they are overreacting, perhaps due to their own

desire for validation (such as the team member who, after another teammate was visibly distressed about a client, said, "You shouldn't be so
upset! You didn't have half as bad a week as me!"), or team members
who have difficulty tolerating others' intense emotion ("Bring it down a
notch, it's not that bad!"), or team members who are more generally emotionally vulnerable and invalidate anything anyone says due to general
irritability. We have experienced eye rolls; muttering under one's breath
("Here we go again!"); deep, audible sighs; and many more behaviors that
communicate invalidation to teammates. The team can try a variety of
strategies, including highlighting such behavior, giving direct feedback,
and assessing what is setting off the behavior as well as its function. Typically, if the team can address the function, the invalidation will die down.
For example, we worked with a clinician who invalidated others' sadness
because the emotion made him uncomfortable. The team made an effort
to expose this person to sadness in team, and to coach him about how to
respond when he felt uncomfortable (saying, "I'm uncomfortable" instead
of "Don't feel so sad!"). If these solutions do not help, the team must consider whether the team member is invalidating clients in session as well;
it may be that further education or supervision about validation more
broadly is needed.

Teams may also have members who invalidate themselves chronically. Team members can highlight this behavior any time they see it.
Contingency management may be particularly helpful: (1) light punishment or lack of reinforcement for the invalidation (e.g., "Hey, you're
really invalidating yourself"), (2) highlight the contingencies (e.g., the
team tells the provider they will pause discussion of the problem until
the invalidation is dealt with: "Let's get you to validate yourself a little
more, then we'll get to problem solving"), and (3) a lot of reinforcement
for self-validation (be sure to know what functions as reinforcement for
this individual: praise, getting more or less attention, or other responses).
This process can be done with a great deal of warmth and compassion.
Reminding team members that they work tirelessly to change this behavior with clients, yet are not embodying this behavior themselves, can be
helpful as well.

A Teammate Dominates the Team Meeting

Many teams we have consulted with have described difficulties with a
member who dominates the team. This style can take a variety of forms.

For example, some team members want to be sure the team has all the details before solving, so they describe the background in too much detail; in this case, using the structure of the agenda, stating clearly what each team member needs during the allotted time, and using a timer will likely help significantly. Some team members share personal information or details that are not relevant to clinical care. In teams with ample time, this may not be a problem, but often it will interfere with others getting sufficient time on the agenda. A simple reminder from the observer, meeting leader, team leader, or any other member, then returning to the agenda, typically resolves this type of problem.

Other times talking a lot is due to a higher level of expertise and/or experience than other teammates possess. It is inevitable that teams in certain settings will have a broad range of expertise. Both of our teams have more and less experienced individuals on the same team: MML's team has the treatment developer and several students with little clinical experience, and JS's team has individuals with decades of experience along with individuals very new to DBT. This dynamic can result in new individuals hesitating to talk, and experienced individuals teaching, correcting, and feeling pressure to control the outcome. It is helpful for more experienced members to share their wisdom and experience with newer members; it can be essential in some situations to have experienced clinicians guide other members. Particularly when one or a few members know DBT better than others, they may need to provide more direct instruction to less experienced members. Ironically, however, it is not always ideal for experts to act like experts. The danger is the team will come to treat this individual as a consultant, rather than an active member of the team. In other words, the team could ask questions and wait for the expert to answer, and take that answer without questioning. This does not fit with the DBT team culture, in which everyone is expected to be active, with all members looking for what is being left out, and the idea that a helpful solution can come from any member. It is essential that the individual with expertise is also challenged if needed, other perspectives are considered, nonexpert opinions are valued, and all members remain very active in problem solving and following the team agreements.

In some teams, it may be difficult to get the expert to shift; they may become distressed if other team members do not follow the expert's advice or do not understand why a certain point is emphasized. Some experienced members are accustomed to being considered the expert in team and may have difficulty letting others provide guidance and suggestions.

Experts can become more forceful, more frustrated, and create distress for teammates as a result. Once again, an open team discussion about making sure *all* team members learn how to become effective team members will be useful. Experts' words of wisdom are extremely important; their ability to teach and model such that others become effective members is equally necessary. The expert can work on stating the point clearly, then letting go, as well as reinforcing others' participation; meanwhile teammates can work on acknowledging the expert's point, searching for the other pole when needed, attending to others' suggestions when useful, and thoughtfully seeking the most skillful way forward.

Certain members may also prefer having a team member who is more active and directive than others, and may reinforce this "expert" style. This is often true with providers who are less experienced, less sure of themselves, or otherwise in need of stronger guidance. If this style is reinforced by the team, it will no longer function as a place where individuals question each other and push each other; it will turn into a place where they only get the one member's opinion, and all the other members become more passive in response.

We worked with a clinician who would only follow the most expert member of the team's consultation, and would take suggestions from her wholesale, regardless of content. The expert member had to move out of the role of team expert (i.e., telling each member how to handle each situation) and start coaching others to provide the feedback, then shaping and strengthening that feedback, in order to bring the team back to its structure. In these situations, an open discussion in team will help lead the team to find effective solutions, targeting both parties' behavior.

Another form of dominance is a "strong personality" in the team, one who interacts with more intensity than the others. Often this is no problem at all, but at certain times it can leave members feeling they have been steamrolled! For example, when a team member is feeling intense guilt about an intervention with a client, a comment that might be intended as irreverent ("Well of course you feel guilty, you screwed up!") might only reinforce the guilt and not move the provider to a more effective, open spot. When a team member is experiencing strong emotion, being highly confrontational may have the opposite of the intended effect. When we have given clinicians feedback in this type of situation, they often respond by saying they are using irreverence, or are "being V6" (i.e., using Level 6 validation, radical genuineness), and therefore don't need to change anything. This, of course, is nondialectical. Irreverence and radical genuineness are both essential in DBT team; in contrast, if such intensity takes the team away from its goals (providing adherent treatment, ensuring feedback is absorbed and implemented, keeping motivation high), it becomes problematic. There may be times when irreverence shuts a teammate down; in such cases, be mindful to notice and address it (rather than think, "That's their problem"). Just as in DBT therapy, we encourage everyone to be their genuine self, *and* to notice when doing so takes the team further from its goals. This is typically less of a problem if confrontation or other irreverence is delivered in a context of a warm, caring team, and more of a problem when teams have tension and a lack of trust. And of course, we do not want anyone to become so frightened to be their "genuine self" that they become quiet; in DBT we speak first, monitor the impact, then move ahead effectively (which might include a simple, "I'm sorry, that wasn't how I intended that comment!"). Over time we expect teammates to become more accustomed to a more direct style of communication.

In cases where the team agrees a change in behavior is needed, and this particular team member continues to dominate time and is not responding to prompts from the team, a stronger intervention may be needed. While the team must be careful not to attack or judge this member, the team or team leader may need to say directly, "This is not useful. We need to ask you to stop," or the leader may discuss the problem with the teammate privately.

A Teammate Talks Too Little

Alternatively, teammates can talk too little. They may be afraid to take up time, hesitant to assert their own opinion, or concerned they don't know enough. Even when providers are early in their career and may not have extensive experience, it is still essential in team that everyone engage in validation, assessment, and problem solving, and that everyone looks for what is left out. Countless times we have seen the least experienced member of the team be the most able to see the other pole; sometimes they are the only one who can see a problem with fresh eyes! When certain members are not speaking, it is useful to put this problem on the agenda to assess what the obstacle is. If this person is simply quiet by nature, there may be no need for change, or just a minor change will help, such as asking them to contribute a small amount each week. If the individual has social anxiety or is otherwise anxious about speaking, or is afraid someone will reject them if they speak up, informal or formal exposure may be useful (e.g., they speak once per team meeting, then observe the team's reactions and note what *actually* happened as a result). The team will hopefully respond in such a way that reduces the anxiety over time. If the team member is not speaking due to frustration with the team, this is an elephant in the room that needs to be discussed. A teammate can ask, "What's going on?" or "How can we help?" We have seen providers stop talking because, according to them, "It makes no difference" or "No one will help me anyway." Reminding the team member of the agreements to speak in team and to keep trying even when frustrated may also be helpful to begin to engage this problem. The team can say, "Shoot, we thought we were being helpful!," then validate, help define, and begin solving the problem. Regardless of the cause, it will be helpful for at least one member, perhaps the observer or team leader, to at times ask this person directly, "What do *you* think?" to ensure that they are actively contributing to the team.

A team member may also neglect to put themselves on the agenda when they actually need help. This is a problem that requires intervention, but may be difficult for the team to identify. Typically, someone on the team will become aware of this person's struggle with a certain client; at this point the team can simply ask why they are not on the agenda (or even tell this person they need to be on the agenda). If the provider repeatedly does not ask for help in team, a more formal assessment may be needed to identify the source of the avoidance. It could be that the provider is already getting their needs met in supervision (in which case the team still may want to know what the issues are), but if the team member is simply not getting any help, due to anxiety, frustration, or other reasons, the team may need to request this person be placed on the agenda, once or over a series of meetings, to address this problem directly.

A Teammate's Fear of Liability Affects Clinical Care

Another common issue is how much the fear of liability can impact team members' behavior. Such fear can lead a provider not only to engage in less effective interventions (e.g., hospitalizing due to fear when this is not the best intervention for the client), but also to be rigid and closed to team suggestions. Ideally, providing the best care makes a team member *less* vulnerable to legal difficulties, but this is not always the case (as in the example above, in which a client is suicidal but hospitalization will reinforce the suicidality; avoiding hospitalization is the most effective path forward but involves some liability risk). When one is fearful about suicide in particular, the team's help is essential to prevent acting from emotion mind (more is said about suicidal clients and the DBT team in Chapter 7).

Fear of liability can be an obstacle for any provider seeing clients with multiple, chronic, severe problems. If one wishes to treat such challenging clients, certain skills will be needed to tolerate this fear and still act effectively. The team's job here is to pay attention and make sure that the team member is trained in the necessary areas to manage the client's problems, is not avoiding, is taking the risk seriously, and is implementing effective, acceptable strategies. The team can provide a "reality check" for these fears by confirming or discounting those fears and helping the team member take effective action. The team member can document this discussion, as well, which may further allay their concerns. In cases where the team notices fear of liability (or any other factors) are interfering with effective care and the team member is unaware of the problem, they call out the elephant in the room and then use a variety of DBT strategies (e.g., commitment strategies, emotion regulation, distress tolerance, and any others that may be helpful) to help their teammate return to effective DBT.

A Teammate Is Too Tight or Too Loose about Adherence

Following the manual to fidelity can be quite challenging at times. This problem can surface in two ways: a team member might follow the manual too tightly, or not follow the manual tightly enough. We have seen many debates in teams about both extremes! And both are problematic. Follow the manual too tightly, and the principles can get lost (Rizvi & Sayrs, in press); idiographic assessment and creative, flexible solutions designed carefully for one particular client are essential components of DBT. DBT was designed to be a highly flexible, principle-driven treatment. If a teammate is responding in a rule-bound way, a discussion of the principles may be very useful, to help the provider see how following rules too closely might actually take the treatment off track.

The term "rigid" is often used when a team member follows the manual in a rule-bound manner. This word may be experienced as judgmental, so the team will also need to define the problem carefully, avoiding any pejorative language. Phrasing such as "It seems like you are trying to follow a rule, but I wonder what the principle here is?" can work; a more careful definition will likely also be needed. Generating multiple solutions is also useful, to help facilitate flexible responding. The team can help orient the teammate to the goal of flexible thinking. Lightly asking, "Are you thinking there's only one solution?" or "Are you worried we are straying from the manual when we discuss other solutions?" may be useful. Focusing on the validity of both poles will be helpful: there are valid reasons why one team member is holding on to one particular solution, and there are valid reasons why other team members are pushing for more flexibility. Highlighting both poles will help move the team toward a synthesis. For example, the team member may feel strongly that their client must enter the skills group immediately in order to learn skills (following a "rule" that all clients must be in a skills group can be ineffective for certain clients); the rest of the team may suggest that the client is not going to learn well in a group. The synthesis could be a few weeks of individual skills training to help a very socially anxious client prepare before entering the highly anxiety-provoking skills group (focusing on the principle of increasing the client's capability by teaching them skills in some format).

Equally challenging is when a team member is not following the manual closely enough. A team member may return to nonbehavioral language, or say the manual is too rigid, or have strong urges to rely on clinical intuition instead of data. This can create tense moments in team, when team members are very attached to doing things "their way," while the rest of the team is concerned but unsure how to proceed. In such a case, it is essential to first call out the elephant in the room, ("I think you are missing something here"), then give a rationale for returning to the manual. The rationale should tie the intervention to the client's and provider's goals, rather than "because the manual says so." For example, we worked with a clinician who typically skipped multiple "core" skills in the emotion regulation module. This particular person did not see their relevance, and wanted to spend more time on the skills he liked and understood. Trying to address this issue was challenging because he was willful about the team's feedback. The team first identified the problem, and asked, "What's the threat?" in other words, what is generating such a strong reaction when the team provides suggestions? This discussion revealed that the provider could not figure out why these skills were even included in the manual. If the team responded with, "You should do this because this is the treatment, it's part of the skills curriculum," it would have landed flat! Instead, the team demonstrated the use of these skills, and how they tied in well with the client's target behaviors. After this illustration, the provider left team enthusiastic about having new ideas for the upcoming session. Such discussions won't always go so smoothly or quickly, but helping the team member see the rationale is important in increasing willingness.

Perhaps the most difficult problem with adherence is when a team identifies a teammate who is not following the manual to fidelity, and the teammate believes they are adherent. This may occur in a team that does not have someone experienced in DBT, or in a team with very experienced members who are unaware they have drifted from the manual. This can be an emotional discussion, where a team member could become defensive because they believe they are providing the best care possible. Remaining dialectical, defining very specifically which behaviors may be problematic (rather than stating globally that a team member is not adherent), and exploring the issue nonjudgmentally are all essential. For example, we (JS) worked with a clinician who readily placed clients on vacations whenever she became frustrated; when the team highlighted that there were other strategies for therapy-interfering behavior, the provider became more polarized and stuck. The team had to focus on very specific examples, relying on the treatment manuals, examples, and extensive validation to guide the discussion. In this case, the team member's frustration decreased and her willingness increased as her skill with additional DBT strategies improved. The team may also benefit from an expert consultation, if unable to resolve the issue with these strategies.

A Teammate Becomes Burned Out

When one member of a team is experiencing burnout, it affects the entire team. Burned-out providers can be less empathic, more judgmental, more irritable, and less creative. After working with many providers over multiple years, we have learned a few important lessons about burnout. First, the term "burnout" requires a behavioral definition from the individual. Despite frequent use of the term, different team members may have very different meanings for this term. For some, burnout is a serious, pervasive condition from which they don't ever really recover; others use it to refer to mild frustration with one particular client. It is important to assess what team members mean when they say they are "burned out." Be sure to ask about any particular situations that set off states of burnout, related emotions, thoughts, and any avoidance of situations/emotions/thoughts to get a clear understanding of what the team member is experiencing.

For example, at one point in my (JS) career, I became burned out. I was afraid of the feeling, so I did not assess carefully at first; I only knew that I had thoughts about hating my career and feeling unwilling to continue. Fortunately, with behavioral and mindfulness training, at some point my team and I realized I needed to define my problem more specifically. I completed a mood record (specifically, I completed the Activity-and-Mood Monitoring Chart; Addis & Martell, 2004, p. 176) daily for several weeks. This helped me define the problem and see how my mood shifted throughout the days and weeks. I was able to narrow in on a brief period, one day each week, when certain administrative duties inevitably caused me high distress. I was so relieved! I realized I did not hate my whole career, I hated one duty, but the thoughts and emotions were spreading throughout the week. With my team's help, I chose One Thing in the Moment as my solution; I acknowledged my distress on that one particular day, and tried to rejoice on other days that I did not have to attend to that task. My point is that carefully defining what is causing distress, and trying to solve that issue while noticing that other elements of one's job/life are pleasant, can reduce that generalized feeling of burnout. This assessment and intervention led me to stop saying "I'm burned out," and instead I said, "I hate one particular hour on Mondays!"

Another important lesson we learned about burnout is the team cannot actually solve burnout. The team can help in a number of ways, including validation, problem solving, phone coverage, even walking someone's dog or buying groceries for them. But placing the burden of solving this state of mind on the team can lead to unrealistic expectations and active passivity from the team member. The team member must be willing to acknowledge their distress to the team, be open to their feedback, and be willing to work on solutions. We worked with a clinician who came to team, placed herself on the agenda, and said she was burned out. The team was very concerned and really rallied, trying to assess and offer solutions. For several weeks thereafter, the provider said, "I'm still burned out. Your solutions weren't enough," and became increasingly demoralized and hopeless. We realized this team member was not taking any ownership of her distress; instead, she was placing it on the agenda and waiting for relief to happen. We agreed in hindsight that the team had reinforced the notion that the team could solve her burnout. Remember, the team provides consultation, suggestions, and feedback, but does not move in and fix burnout or any other problem; the team member must do this. Had the team started the conversation with this mindset, the team member may have been pushed to try more solutions, assess for herself, and directly wrestle with the causes of her distress.

If the solutions aren't working, just as in therapy, teams can look for problems such as gaps in the clinician's understanding (more assessment is needed), willfulness, whether the solutions are aimed at the right problems, and so on. Some problems may be beyond what a team can solve. It will be important not to harm the entire team in an effort to save one team member; the leader may need to intervene, and/or an outside source of help may be needed if the team's ideas are not helpful. Ultimately, certain team members' motivation may dwindle over time. We have seen many people eagerly do DBT with very difficult clients for a few years, then decide they are ready for something new, or something less intense and stressful. While doing their best to problem-solve in team, radical acceptance is also important. This individual may benefit from a vacation, or at times from ending their membership on the team entirely. On very rare occasions, the team may even suggest a vacation when the team member does not want to stop; this is very infrequent and only done when other interventions don't work, and the burnout is affecting client care. This topic was discussed further in Chapter 3.

Problems That Occur with the Team as a Whole

The team as a whole may also develop problems, where the entire team's culture drifts from the agreements, or a subset of team members may behave problematically. All of the above principles remain relevant, but the team may also want to consider additional solutions, such as:

1. Define the problem together, as a team.
2. Review the team agreements together.
3. Use exercises, free-writes, discussions, and retreats to change the norms and culture in the team, and help everyone move toward effective solutions.
4. Change the structure of the team as needed, such as by adding to observer reminders in order to address particular behaviors, or setting aside time to discuss team problems on a regular basis.

5. Brainstorm ways teammates can reinforce the desired behaviors. Keep in mind that bringing up the problem is only the first step; the team will need to be mindful of reinforcing discussions of elephants in the room without reinforcing a culture of complaining without solutions. Effective identification of problems, assessment, and solutions should be carefully and deliberately reinforced.

Some examples of team problems are discussed below. As mentioned previously, these are only a few of many possible solutions; teams will need to assess and develop solutions that fit their particular problems.

The Team Is Not Validating Each Member Sufficiently

We have worked with teams that lean heavily on the change side, and run short on validation. There will be many situations where this is not a problem; the team is often resilient and can quickly offer solutions without much validation. There may be times, however, when the team feels less resilient, or a teammate is especially emotional about a particular client. Teammates can remain mindful of how much the team searches for the kernel of truth, conveys that a teammate's reactions make sense, and overall accepts them exactly where they are at. The observer can ask the team at the end of the meeting whether everyone was mindful of validating each other. The team can also ask specific members if they received enough validation to keep their motivation high, and of course any individual member should ask for more validation if needed.

The Team Avoids Pushing for Change

Teams might avoid change for a variety of reasons. For example, a team's discomfort with intense emotion might mean they reinforce distracting from a difficult issue or particular strategy, or avoiding a topic altogether. The team may validate extensively and tell members their strategies were effective when they were not. On a more subtle level, teams can inadvertently reinforce those who express contentment and punish those who express problems in team, which can build a culture of apparent competence and disingenuousness.

Remaining aware of the contingencies at play will be essential. When a team member expresses unhappiness, a particular difficulty, or a need for change in team, the response that individual receives will determine whether they discuss a need for change again. As stated above, it will be essential to reinforce the team member, even if the topic is uncomfortable or painful. Becoming defensive, arguing, or invalidating a team member will *decrease* the likelihood of further problem identification and solution, whereas listening, problem solving, and validating will likely *increase* the probability of this effective behavior. Knowing what would function as a reinforcer for this individual, and delivering the reinforcer even if one is hurt or frustrated, is a difficult skill to acquire. Being extremely mindful of one's reactions during these conversations can facilitate open and honest discussions.

At the same time, teams will need to be aware of shaping team members into complaining; the reinforcement should be aimed at productive, constructive discussion and problem solving. Unproductive complaints, or emphasis only on problems and not on solutions, will be just as damaging to team culture as staying silent. Having team discussions and mindfully reinforcing effective team behavior are the strategies that will help the team move toward a more effective culture. For example, if a teammate says, "You guys are in a bad mood today!" the team can request a more specific restatement, such as "I feel really invalidated right now" (an effective description of how they feel). At this point, instead of acting on the urge to say, "But we just validated you!" it will be more effective for the team to pause, listen, find the validity, and say, "Shoot, that's the opposite of our intention! Can you tell us exactly what we said that felt invalidating?" This will likely both reinforce effective behavior and lead to a helpful solution.

A variety of strategies can be used to facilitate a focus on change. First, teams can practice giving each other difficult feedback, even feedback that is not true and provided solely for practice. For example, in our team, we practiced telling each other we had body odor, simply to practice saying something difficult to, and receiving difficult feedback from, a teammate. This is a very useful exercise because it develops the repertoire of saying and hearing something uncomfortable, where everyone practices at once. As mentioned previously, teams can also consider using shaping, where the team practices increasingly difficult and close-to-home topics, gradually building the intensity until teammates are accustomed to hearing feedback about real behaviors. Discussing afterward can help the team give feedback to each other; if this exercise moves into language that is hurtful, mean-spirited, or judgmental, the team can then discuss whether and how to shape that behavior.

The Team Does Not Get through the Agenda

Not having time to address high-priority items on the agenda repeatedly, across different team members and problems, is typically either a structural problem where the team is not using the agenda in an effective way, and/or due to teammates struggling with getting members to stop talking when their turn ends. For the first problem, having a team discussion about the agenda will be useful. This discussion may lead to ideas including increased structure, the use of a timer to indicate the end of each person's turn, and focused requests for specific help. If the team is struggling with getting people to stop talking, the team can practice telling someone it's time to stop (everyone role-plays this prompt), and practice stopping speaking midsentence. These exercises will help members be more aware of how they interfere with the structure of the team when they continue talking after their turn is up, and/or when they allow others to keep talking after their turn. Once again, reviewing the rationale for such a structure can help too; for example, discussing the impact of one member going over time means that two other members don't get their time can help increase the mindfulness and willingness of the team to address the problem. The team can also remind each other that each team member just needs enough to get through the week, and the entire problem does not need to be fully defined nor solved by the end of the team meeting. With the challenging problems our clients present, it is not reasonable to expect to solve everything in one team meeting! Finally, if this is an ongoing problem, the team may consider lengthening the team meeting. It may be there truly is not enough time to meet the needs of the team and clients, in which case adding more time may be a straightforward solution.

Outsiders and Insiders

Teams can become divided between those with "insider status" and those with "outsider status," or members who feel like they are an outsider in the team. This can happen in a variety of ways, with respect to race/ethnicity/culture, age, supervisor/supervisee status, friendships, and many other roles. We have seen this problem deeply divide teams, where certain individuals feel excluded and misunderstood. In our experience, this problem is significantly worse when it is an elephant in the room; outsider status often needs to be talked about openly. We have helped teams discuss problems around religion (one member feeling discriminated against in team based on comments about religion), race (several members experienced comments by a team member as racist), gender (actions taken by one member were experienced as discriminatory by several members of the team), sexual orientation (one member felt discriminated against as the team's only lesbian), and so on. We have seen these problems arise in so many teams we are convinced they are nearly universal.

This type of situation is difficult because it is often not openly discussed. One solution is to conduct an exercise in team, either a discussion and/or a free-write exercise, focusing on ways each member feels like an outsider, in general and in team. This may highlight ways the team can become more aware of the experiences of each team. In our team, none of us realized some of the phrases we used were offensive to one team member until we had a discussion about what events in team made each person feel separated and excluded. It was easy for the team to acknowledge what had happened (the fallibility agreement) and stop making those comments, once they were made aware, but it did not come to light until we had a discussion in team.

This also highlights the importance of each team member using distress tolerance. To completely avoid saying things that rub team members the wrong way is impossible! And if the team slows down and discusses every single one, there will be no time to work on providing excellent clinical care. Little problems in team discussion can be addressed quickly, but more in-depth discussions about outsider status might work well if they are scheduled, perhaps once per year, so the issue is addressed regularly but does not overtake other, equally important topics.

Observer Feedback Is Aversive

This is an easy problem to slip into because the observer is primarily focused on identifying problems and moving the team toward change, which can, over time, become frustrating to teammates. In such a case, it may be helpful to review the team agreements and the reason why these agreements are important. This review can help everyone remember the rationale for the observer role, and why that role is so essential; this also helps everyone remember that the observer is not out to punish everyone, but to bring the team's attention to moments when someone strays from the agreements. Emphasizing the importance of developing behaviors that support team culture, even when the feedback may be difficult to hear, also will help maintain the observer's effectiveness. When teams regularly rotate roles, all team members have the experience of being the observer and are more likely to appreciate the difficulty of the role. This can lead to more gratitude and less frustration when the observer calls out a particular behavior. If a team member is defensive when the observer provides feedback, highlight the defensiveness. If it warrants further attention, place this individual on the agenda and discuss the problem as a team. Teams may discuss how to give feedback, and even practice doing so, to help team members become less sensitive and better able to absorb observer feedback. And finally, share the responsibility of monitoring the team with all members. Instead of relying on just the observer, remind team members that *everyone* monitors and alerts the team. We have worked with teams where all members remained silent when there was a problem in team, assuming the observer would catch it and manage it. This can result in problems being missed, as well as a lot of passivity among team members. Expecting all members to take responsibility for the culture in every team will help address these problems. In our (JS) team, we encouraged this tendency by adding 5 minutes at the end of team, where the observer reads each of the reminders and asks the team if they noticed those problems occurring (see Chapter 4 for a description). Team members thoughtfully answer and discuss any problems that may have arisen (e.g., one member might state that he was distracted by a text at a certain point in team). Solutions may be discussed, or the team member/topic can be placed on the agenda for the following team meeting. Adding this brief discussion to the end of the team meeting briefly engages the entire team in the discussion of team culture each week, and provides a system for catching behaviors that the observer might have missed. It also allows an opportunity for team members to be reinforced for maintaining team culture (e.g., "Aisha helped us to be more dialectical today. Nice job!"), and provides a useful training opportunity as well, in which trainees can learn from comments made by more experienced members.

The Team Is Too Large or Too Small

Teams can become too large. There are few rules about how large or small a DBT team should be. As will be discussed further in Chapter 8, at least two people must be present to be a team, and the upper limit is based on effectiveness—making sure the team functions to help every member provide the best DBT possible. Identifying the point at which the size of the team has become problematically large can be very challenging. There may be subtle signs of dissatisfaction, such as comments about needing more time, not getting needs met, or not knowing each other well enough to feel comfortable being vulnerable. Having regular check-ins about the health of the team and how everyone is doing can help pinpoint when size becomes an issue for the team. As mentioned in a previous example, my (JS) team expressed dissatisfaction, which prompted a series of extended discussions and exercises and ultimately the decision to divide the team into two separate teams. This was a difficult decision because our teammates really liked each other and did not want to be separated. When we split the team, we scheduled the two team meetings back-to-back, with a 30-minute overlap so everyone could eat lunch together and we could address items that concerned everyone (e.g., brief coordination of care, updates, announcements).

Even more difficult is when some members of team believe it's too large, and others do not want to change the format. This can become a challenge for the team leader; assessing exactly what needs are not being met and brainstorming multiple solutions to address those problems may help resolve them without splitting up the team. For example, if one person wants more time because they prefer to have an extended period to talk about their clinical work, it may be more helpful to work with this individual to change their expectations (e.g., rarely will they get a full 30 minutes for their own agenda items), make sure they have regular contact with teammates outside of team, and validate their wish to have much more time in team. If all other members of the team are fine with the size of the team, these solutions may be sufficient.

Teams can also be too small; we have worked with teams of two people, and in some cases this works very well. If two people are struggling to maintain a dialectical stance, becoming polarized rather than searching for and finding what is being left out, it is possible another person or two may help diversify the opinions and strategies in team. The team can discuss their effectiveness and whether they have enough people to generate multiple solutions and avoid becoming polarized.

The Team Is Affected by One Problematic Member

We have seen several teams significantly impacted by one particular member of the team. This member might not be respected or liked, or frustrate everyone else. We have seen examples of one member refusing to follow the agreements, or coming back with pejorative comments when other teammates are vulnerable. This member may be nondialectical, judgmental, or nonbehavioral. We have also seen teams respond to one individual differently than anyone else for no obvious reason. Behavioral specificity will be essential: the problem should not be described as, "I just don't mesh well with him" or "She's not even doing DBT"; instead, if the team can focus on the behavior not the person, and work toward a clear definition of the problem, with examples, it will be easier to get down to the business of solving the problem. For example, a team member might say, "Your irreverence often hurts my feelings" or "I start to feel helpless when you tell us each of our suggestions won't work" or "I notice that when you provide suggestions, you often blend DBT with other treatments that seem contradictory to me. I find I get confused. Would you provide suggestions from one consistent theoretical orientation?" Giving teammates difficult feedback is not easy, and teammates will need to remain mindful to avoid having their frustration make the situation worse. During this conversation, remaining dialectical, finding the validity in both poles, being compassionate and empathic, and remaining behaviorally specific will hopefully help the team look at the problem with curiosity and interest.

Once again, the team will need to determine if the problem is worth solving. If it is not interfering with members' motivation and capability, it may be possible to just let it lie. For example, we worked with a team with one member who made shocking comments that were meant to be irreverent, but for many teammates crossed the line into offensive. After calling out the elephant that many members were feeling angry after several of these comments, and a discussion about how this person did not intend for nor realize these comments were offensive, the team decided they would prefer to work on client care, and chose to tolerate these comments. They considered the prioritization of team issues, and decided this person's verbalizations did not rise above the need to address therapy for the therapist. Given the nature of intense group work, tolerating individual differences is often a useful solution in DBT team, allowing such problems to remain a low priority.

At times, one member is problematic because they did not enter the team voluntarily. They may have been forced to join the team by their agency, for example. In addition to the team interventions, this may require the leader to interact with administration, to help them understand the impact of having a reluctant member on the team, and strategize for how to increase willingness and/or avoid adding individuals to the team without a commitment process. The leader may also have a frank conversation with this individual, highlighting or reviewing what is expected of each team member.

Unfortunately, as discussed in the chapter on the team leader (Chapter 3), there may be times when a team member is simply not a good fit, and their behavior becomes a high priority for the team. Someone who makes fun of the team agreements, or is judgmental of teammates despite repeated feedback, or is burned out and does not want to work on this issue, or does not want to do DBT, may simply be a poor match for the team. The leader and the team can make attempts to solve the problem, but sometimes this will end with an individual departing from the team, by their own choice or, more rarely, by the team leader's choice. While this withdrawal or removal can be upsetting, we have seen clear examples where this was the best solution for everyone. Much as in DBT treatment, this solution should be treated as a last resort, after all others have failed.

There Is No Identified Primary Provider for a Client

When there is disagreement within the team about which clinician should be functioning as the primary provider for a given client, the integrity of the treatment can be threatened. In DBT, the individual therapist is typically the primary provider. It is the primary provider, along with the client, who develops the treatment plan, manages the client's suicide risk, and monitors progress through treatment.

There are some exceptions, of course; for example, when the client does not have an individual therapist (e.g., is only attending skills group). In such cases, clearly delineating who is making treatment decisions with the client, who carries clinical responsibility, and who addresses suicide risk and other life-threatening behaviors will be essential. If the client has an individual therapist outside of the DBT team/agency, there may be additional issues to deal with, particularly if that person is not providing individual DBT. The division of clinical tasks will need to be clear; for example, the team will want to be sure the client's outside provider completes paperwork to document who carries responsibility (see Linehan, 2015b, for a sample agreement for the outside provider to complete). If there is no outside provider, the team leader will need to make sure that the skills trainer is aware of this fact and understands the role, and inform the team of inclusion/exclusion decisions (e.g., many programs will not allow clients at high suicide risk into their skills training group if there is no individual therapist to assess and address that risk) such that the client gets the best care possible.

In other teams, we have seen DBT team psychiatrists struggle with these roles. Psychiatrists are often accustomed to being the lead provider, due to their training and working in other settings where this is the norm. Psychiatrists also often bear more liability, so may have a strong desire to make clinical decisions. The DBT principle that the individual therapist is the primary therapist may cause confusion and frustration for a psychiatrist joining a DBT team. Prevention strategies will be important in such cases; the psychiatrist must understand before joining the team that the individual therapist will serve as the primary therapist and generate the treatment plan with the client; the psychiatrist, skills trainer, and others are "hired on" by the individual therapist and client. This does not change their role with the client (e.g., psychiatrists still provide medication management as they typically would); it simply means the individual therapist is considered the primary driver of the treatment. In other settings, the agency itself will interfere with this structure; the team leader may then need to address this issue with the administration. Returning to the importance of providing evidence-based care (including outcomes, cost-effectiveness, and liability) often helps make this case (see Chapter 3 for a discussion of interacting with administration).

The Team Disagrees about Prioritization

Perhaps most difficult of all is when one or more team members see a significant team or provider problem, and others in team do not want to spend team time on it. They may not see it as a problem themselves, or have other issues they see as higher priority, or do not want to engage in a challenging discussion. This is a difficult dialectic; on the one hand, if one team member is distressed, the team will try to take that problem very seriously, search for the validity in that position, and work to solve it. That individual can use time on the agenda to work on their own distress in team, which may involve change on the part of the individual and/or the team. On the other hand, other teammates' need for time is important too. It will be equally important for every member to remember that all team members are doing the very best they can, and that many issues in team will go unaddressed. The team leader may need to help navigate whether a problem rises to the level of being a problem for the entire team, remains something that an individual can deal with during their own turn on the agenda, or falls into the category of something the team chooses not to address.

Conclusion

This chapter focused on some of the many problems that can arise in a DBT team, which, if not addressed, can threaten the team's well-being. While it is true that DBT teams can run into some truly difficult interpersonal problems, it is also true that the team has tremendous wisdom. Openly discussing the problems and letting the entire team tackle them, as a team, can result in incredibly helpful solutions, and the team can grow and bond as a result. Remember, these are people that were selected for the team because they are dedicated to DBT, the clients, and the team itself. They know DBT skills and strategies, and know how to apply them to themselves and others. The key is to set up the culture such that these problems can be brought into the open in an effective way by remaining dialectical, behaviorally specific, nonjudgmental, and focused on emotion. With the guidance and structure provided by the agreements and the team leader, the team will find ways through these difficulties that are creative, compassionate, and wise.

IDEAS FOR PRACTICE

- Arrange a retreat for your team.
- Have a discussion about one of the team check-in prompts (see pages 125–126, or one you create that is tailored specifically to your team).
- Complete a formal assessment of burnout or any other relevant topic. Each member shares their answers. The team then discusses similarities, differences, and challenges the team may face as a result.
- Discuss recent team-interfering behavior that each team member engaged in. Keep the focus on your own behavior. Describe for the team what led up to the behavior and what might be maintaining it. Ask for help assessing and solving the problem.
- Identify whether each team member tends to avoid tension or conflict in team or address it directly. Discuss when this tendency is effective and when it is not; brainstorm ways to build skills for the other pole

(e.g., if one member tends to avoid addressing team problems, they might practice Opposite Action and DEAR MAN; if another member tends to react more strongly than other teammates to team tension, they might practice Radical Acceptance and Nonjudgmentally).

- Rotate the role of being "the team expert" or having a more dominant style for an entire team meeting. In this exercise, each team member will get a chance to be more active and directive for a team meeting, while the rest of the team practices sitting back and being less directive. This can highlight each team member's natural tendency and help each member try out different styles. After each member has had a turn, have a team discussion about what was noticed and how this could help team interactions in the future.

- As a team, review Chapter 1. Assess whether the team has drifted away from practices that help maintain the DBT team culture. Use the Problem Solving skill to implement solutions.

- Have a team discussion about where you would like your team to be in 1 year. What changes would you like to see? Set reasonable targets for specific behavior change the team can start implementing immediately, to work toward those goals.

Suicide Risk and the DBT Team

One of the most difficult events a team may deal with is the death of a client, and particularly death by suicide. While this is a rare event, over the course of a career it is likely that most clinicians will be impacted by suicide in some way. Due to its infrequency, clinicians may be unprepared emotionally, and not have strategies in place to deal with the often intense impact of a client suicide. Some team members will have no history with suicide, and may not know what to expect; other clinicians may have previous, personal and/or professional, experience with suicide that can result in strong and even unexpected reactions. Clinicians may also have a tendency to avoid this topic, due to the intense emotions such discussions can create. Teams will benefit from establishing strategies for before, during, and in the aftermath of a suicide crisis, because intense emotion and fast-moving events can interfere with wise mind decision making. Many of the topics included here will also apply to other clinical crises, such as nonsuicidal self-injury, nonlethal suicide behavior, and the death of a client by homicide or accident. This chapter focuses on suicide risk with respect to DBT team only; guidance for managing suicide risk, within DBT or more broadly, can be found elsewhere (e.g., Linehan, 1993; Katz & Korslund, in press; Sung, 2016a, 2016b; *suicidology.org*; *sprc. org*; *intheforefront.org*). This chapter is expressly *not* written to provide legal advice; if legal liability for a suicide is a concern, we recommend contacting one's malpractice carrier, whose recommendations may take priority over the suggestions provided here.

Before a Suicide Crisis

There are steps for a DBT team to take before a crisis, including establishing structure, attending trainings, developing procedures, and engaging in exercises that help the team prepare.

Establishing Structure

When working with high-risk clients, the DBT team can provide essential structure to try to prevent suicide, in both the immediate sense and over the long term. In particular, DBT teams can use the team agenda to prevent and proactively address such crises. The team agenda can provide structure in the following ways:

- A reminder to discuss team members' work with high-risk clients. The meeting leader can read reminders to the team to place oneself on the agenda when one or more clients are engaging in risky behavior or doing worse in therapy. The team as a whole will remain constantly vigilant about the management of high-risk clients.

- A reminder to use a risk assessment form. The meeting leader can also assess and provide reminders for team members' paperwork completion. Ensuring each member is regularly assessing for risk and completing risk assessments and documentation (e.g., the LRAMP; Linehan, Comtois, & Ward-Ciesielski, 2012) when risk is heightened can increase the likelihood that providers will monitor and intervene effectively.

- A prioritization system for team discussion that emphasizes high-risk situations, focusing on each team member's capability and motivation to intervene effectively. The team will assess and address any obstacles to providing the best care possible in these situations. Obstacles may include provider fear, frustration, avoidance, skills deficit, or a variety of other issues; the team can generate and facilitate the use of effective interventions to benefit both the provider and the client(s).

- A reminder to plan video/audio recordings of sessions. Teams that monitor each other's work via reviewing video/audio recordings of sessions may be more likely to help each other notice and address crises earlier in their development.

- Overall, the DBT team helps monitor and facilitate team members' effective strategies, which help minimize suicide risk. This includes making sure each provider directly assesses risk, actively manages risk, does not avoid the topic or particular clients, and documents these activities in a timely manner.

Attending Trainings

All team members should attend training in assessing and managing suicide risk from an expert in the field. After obtaining basic training, one or more team members can attend additional trainings on a regular basis and bring the information back to the team. This will help the team become aware of the most recent developments and be able to respond even more effectively to situations related to suicide. Ensuring the training is based on relevant data (as opposed to just the trainer's personal experience) will be important in obtaining the most helpful, evidence-based information.

Developing Procedures

Teams will benefit from thoughtfully developing procedures to follow in the event of a suicide, and to have these prepared prior to any suicide crisis. Sung (2016a, 2016b) has prepared a detailed set of recommendations teams may use to develop their own procedures pertaining to client suicide, including tasks to complete immediately after a suicide, addressing emotional responses to the suicide, and conducting a case review. We recommend teams carefully tailor these recommendations to their own particular setting, to ensure that the team discusses and comes to a shared understanding of how these situations will be handled. If teams already have a procedure for managing a client's death by suicide, they may wish to review these procedures regularly, and read others' protocols (such as the citations provided here) to be sure they have included all of the necessary steps. Because these situations are often extremely emotional, and can at times become litigious, careful thought and team discussion, in advance, can help to prevent additional difficulties in a time of crisis.

Engaging in Exercises

Teams may also benefit from engaging in exercises pertaining to managing suicide and high-risk behaviors, which may help team members better predict and understand their own and each other's responses and thereby minimize fear-based clinical decisions. They can also increase motivation and dedication to this difficult work. Openly discussing values and emotions related to suicide before a crisis is extremely helpful in preparing providers and a team for suicide-related crises.

Two examples of team exercises are included below; teams should also consider creating exercises that are more tailored to their particular needs. Certain team members may have a very strong reaction to these exercises, encompassing a wide range of emotions. This may be particularly true if a team member has experienced the suicide of a loved one or a client in the past, but they may also cause strong emotion in those who have never been directly touched by suicide. Team members can validate extensively; it is important to avoid conveying that high levels of emotion are problematic. Any communication of disapproval during this exercise may punish the expression of emotion and requests for help. If team members believe they must hide certain beliefs or reactions, they may not ask for assistance before, during, or after high-risk situations. Validation levels 4 (this makes sense given your history) and 5 (this makes sense given the current circumstances) may be particularly helpful.

Exercise 1*

The first exercise includes questions that prompt team members to explore their values and belief systems about the nature and meaning of death and suicide, as well as their beliefs about their own role in trying to stop suicide. These questions are meant to be open-ended, encouraging exploration of how one's values may influence decisions made in therapy and with each other in team.

Team members quietly write the answers to these questions:

- "What is death?"
- "What are my beliefs about suicide?"
- "Do my clients have a right to kill themselves?"
- "Do I have a right to stop them?"
- "Do I have a right to kill myself?"
- "Does anyone have the right to stop me?"

---

*Adapted with permission from Marsha M. Linehan, unpublished, University of Washington Behavioral Research and Therapy Clinics.

Team members then share their answers. They do not discuss each response until everyone has shared. This discussion may occur across several team meetings, but for the initial discussion leave at least 15 minutes.

Once each member has shared, the team may begin a discussion of the implications of members' responses. For example, the team may discuss one member's belief that suicide is immoral, and how this value system may impact the team member's behavior in high-risk situations. At the other pole, a teammate may believe clients do have the right to kill themselves, and they do not have the right to stop them. This belief system will also have significant impact on the provider's behavior. Team members' religious/spiritual beliefs, cultural practices, past experience with suicide, and any other relevant factors can be included. What dialectics arise in this discussion? How do each member's beliefs and values impact their implementation of DBT? The aim is not to identify "right" or "wrong" perspectives, nor to change or "fix" anyone's perspective; it is merely to become aware of tendencies and vulnerabilities in advance. The team can then brainstorm solutions, with respect to particular clients or across clients. This might include writing out steps to help each team member remain effective when in emotion mind, or agreements about how the individual and team will notice when one has strayed from best practices in these situations.

For example, for a period of time after my dear friend died from cancer, I (JS) noticed I felt angry at my clients when they considered suicide, and had frequent thoughts such as "It's not fair to purposefully take your life when others die without wanting to." While this reaction made perfect sense, my team helped me see the potential for me to be in emotion mind and therefore less effective with my suicidal clients. The conversations I had with the team did not remove those thoughts, but gave me and the entire team more awareness, and helped me to bring the issue up regularly until my grieving became less intense.

Exercise 2*

This exercise is based on the Cope Ahead skill (Linehan, 2015a, 2015b) and can be easily adapted to meet any team's specific needs. It

---

*Adapted with permission from Marsha M. Linehan, unpublished, University of Washington Behavioral Research and Therapy Clinics.

is particularly useful for team members who experience intense emotion when dealing with high-risk clients. Once again, in this exercise, team members write out their own answers without comment; discussion takes place after all members have completed written answers to the first two questions.

1. Write out, using the Describe skill, a situation related to a client's suicidal behavior that prompts intense emotion for you. This situation may be hypothetical, something you worry about happening to you in the future, or something you have experienced in the past that remains upsetting to you. Be specific. What about this scenario is causing the emotion? (For example, providers have reported anticipating such outcomes as a lawsuit after the death of a client, the clinic getting shut down as a result of a client's suicide, experiencing intense guilt and shame, losing the trust of their colleagues, and getting a text that the client is attempting suicide at that moment and being unable to reach them.)

   a. Use the Check the Facts skill; in other words, identify any assumptions, judgments, and biased thinking. How realistic are your fears? Adjust your description as needed.

   b. Name the emotions that would likely occur in this situation.

2. Generate a list of responses that could be effective in that situation. Once again, be specific. Write out in detail how you would cope with the following: the situation, other individuals, your thoughts, your urges, and your emotions.

3. Discuss your fears and strategies with your teammates. Team members can validate and provide additional suggestions for effective responses.

4. Imagine the situation in your mind, as vividly as possible. Doing so is an essential step in the Cope Ahead skill (as opposed to simply thinking about the situation). Imagine experiencing your reaction, including thoughts, emotions, and actions, as if they were occurring in this moment.

5. Then rehearse coping effectively, in your mind. Once again, it is essential not only to decide on a strategy or solution, but to *rehearse* it in your imagination. Remember to rehearse strategies for responding to all of the following that are relevant: the situation, other individuals, your thoughts, your urges, and your emotions. This rehearsal means walking

through all the strategies, detail by detail, in your mind's eye, as if they were occurring in this moment.

6. Imagine what obstacles will occur and what new problems you may face in this situation as you are trying to cope. Again, rehearse coping effectively with each.

7. Discuss this exercise with your teammates. Brainstorm what other obstacles might occur and the best possible responses. Teams can also help to refine solutions if it is difficult to think of an effective response.

In our experience, there is a wide variety of feared or dreaded outcomes, and team members are often unaware of their impact. As a result, clinicians may act out of emotion mind more often when in crisis, and their teammates may invalidate or offer ineffective problem solving. These two exercises can help team members become more mindful of what might influence their behavior. These exercises can be done independently, and also can complement each other; the first exercise draws out team members' more general beliefs about suicide and death, while the second provides an element of exposure to the more difficult aspects of a suicide crisis, along with exploration of solutions while in a calm state. Together, they can help team members understand and react much more effectively. As mentioned above, teams will also benefit from generating their own exercises, tailored to their own challenges.

During a Suicide Crisis

Teams can also be instrumental in supporting its members during a suicide crisis. In DBT, many of our clients regularly experience intense thoughts and urges regarding suicide, and not all suicide thoughts or urges rise to the level of crisis. A suicide crisis is a situation where the provider believes risk is suddenly much higher and the provider and client are unable to reduce the risk in the immediate sense. The client may be unwilling to follow a plan, or the clinician may believe the client does not possess the skill to endure a situation without resorting to very dangerous behavior such as a suicide attempt or risky intentional self-harm. In such a situation, all of the DBT principles and strategies are implemented with the client, just as with any other target (e.g., assessment, commitment strategies, chain analysis, solution analysis, validation, dialectical strategies, etc.); these will not be reviewed here but can be found in Linehan (1993, 2015a, 2015b) and Katz and Korslund (in press). Similarly, all of the team strategies discussed in this book are relevant. We review a few strategies here with a specific focus on suicide, to help the team navigate particularly intense moments in DBT treatment.

1. First and foremost, validate and encourage each other. Not only are suicide and other high-risk crises very stressful, they are also exhausting and time-consuming. Team members will likely need to hear that their reactions make sense, they are doing this for a reason, they are doing all the things they need to do for that client, it is short term, and the team is there to support them. Chocolate, coffee, flowers, and other gestures are also much appreciated in times of crisis!

2. Assess. The team can help identify instances where a team member may need additional help, personally and/or with clients, as well as any obstacles in provider motivation and skill. It will be important for the team to understand, as clearly as possible, where the difficulties lie, so they can validate and problem-solve effectively.

3. Provide coaching. This would include all the strategies discussed in the Therapy for the Therapist chapter (Chapter 5), such as helping the team members(s) tolerate distress, regulate emotions, and get into wise mind, as well as providing practical suggestions for validating, assessing, and intervening with the client. Team members can make sure the therapist is proactively monitoring risk, communicating with the client, and engaging in the situation even when urges to avoid might be strong.

4. Provide coaching outside of team. Having access to team members in the office before and after session, and perhaps more importantly, after hours at any time, is essential in providing excellent care to clients in crisis. Team members can make themselves available at any time a crisis arises for a teammate, to help manage frustration and fear, and to provide suggestions and direct instruction.

5. Provide respite. If a client has been in a prolonged crisis, a team member may experience fatigue. The team can offer a brief break by taking over phone coaching for a weekend, covering for this client and/or other clients while the provider takes a day at the spa, or otherwise helping share the burden during the crisis. This provides the provider with the opportunity to rest and rejuvenate.

6. Provide practical assistance. Team members can also provide practical assistance to help a teammate engage with the client in crisis. If a provider needs to spend more time on the phone, with other team members, or in additional sessions, the team can offer to walk their dog, pick up groceries, provide child care, see their other clients, or absorb other duties, on a temporary basis, to provide the extra bandwidth to deal with the situation.

After a Suicide Crisis

There may be no action needed after a crisis. The client's risk may decrease and the teammate, client, and the whole team may return to business as usual. Alternatively, even if a client pulls through the crisis, a team member may need coaching and help recovering, to avoid ineffectively expressing frustration or exhaustion to the client, or to avoid reinforcing a client's crisis behaviors. Team members may also need assistance in generating a treatment plan to avoid such difficulties in the future.

The DBT team is most needed, however, when a client's increased risk results in death, and particularly death by suicide. Fortunately, it is rare for a client crisis to end in death; however, teams will likely deal with a suicide at some point. The news of a client suicide may come in a variety of ways. A family member may inform the team, or a team member may see it on the news or Internet. The news may come immediately after the death or after a period of time has passed.

Having a plan for how to communicate regarding a client's death may be important for larger teams. Oftentimes, it is not the provider who first learns of the death, but a receptionist or another team member. It will be helpful to delineate in advance whom to notify, including the primary therapist (in most teams this is the individual therapist; in teams not offering individual therapy, this will be the person who was the primary contact for the client), team leader, the entire team, and the agency, if relevant. The means of notification should also be described, including whether individuals should be informed in person, via phone, or via secure e-mail. In our experience, e-mail is the least preferred form, as it can come across as colder and less supportive, and can delay notification unnecessarily. In person is ideal; however, the delay required in waiting to see a person face to face may make this approach less desirable. Phone contact has worked well for us, as it allows the person delivering the news to communicate immediately, convey warmth, and also gauge how much support will be needed.

The primary therapist and team leader should be notified immediately. Together, they can agree on a plan to notify the team. The primary therapist may want to inform everyone on the team, or they may be grateful to have the team leader do this for them. All members of the team are alerted as quickly as possible. It is important to remember that confidentiality continues beyond death, and in some states the cause of death is confidential; this means team members may not inform nonteam members, such as a teacher or family member, of the cause of death in certain cases. Knowing the state laws regarding confidentiality and death in advance is helpful.

It's important to remember that therapists may not know what to do after a suicide, due to lack of experience and/or intense emotion. The team leader may need to provide a lot of support to help the therapist and other team members work through this difficult situation, and in turn, the team leader may need additional support. After learning of the suicide, important issues for the team include: (1) addressing any liability issues; (2) supporting each other; (3) monitoring team functioning; (4) interacting with the family; (5) informing other clients; and 6) finding meaning. These are addressed in turn below.

Liability

The period of time immediately after a suicide can be a very trying time, particularly if one is grieving and simultaneously experiencing guilt or fear one will be blamed for the death. As we have discussed previously, making decisions based on fear of liability can be problematic, and after a suicide that fear may be intense. At times, addressing liability and providing effective clinical care can seem to be in direct opposition. It will not be effective to let fear of liability govern all decisions regarding suicide risk; instead, attempting to remain dialectical, balancing the two demands, will likely be more effective. This means searching for the validity in *both* poles (liability and clinical care), obtaining consultation, and utilizing wise mind in deciding how to move forward.

The chances of legal action are actually low (according to the American Psychological Association, less than 2% of psychologists will experience a malpractice lawsuit in a 20-year career; Novotney, 2016). Taking steps to address liability can be very calming to a frightened team member (and possibly anxiety-provoking to one who does not want to spend time thinking about liability!). After a suicide, team support may be particularly important with respect to liability fears. We discuss liability first not because it is necessarily more important than other topics listed here, but because seeking consultation after a suicide often involves time-sensitive topics and actions, and could influence other steps taken in such situations. Areas for the team to consider with respect to liability include:

- First and foremost, team members can help the teammates who had contact with the client to obtain consultation from the malpractice carrier. The primary therapist or other provider who had clinical responsibility should contact the malpractice carrier upon learning of a suicide. They will likely need to provide information to the carrier to obtain effective consultation; having the team leader or another team member sit with them and even help answer questions may be needed. This step will help catch any issues early, provide structure for how the provider and team proceed, and importantly, soothe fears about liability.

- In this initial consultation, it will be important to discuss what can and cannot be discussed in team. If the suicide is discussed with others, that information may not be considered privileged. Ask the malpractice carrier about these matters (rather than a friend or colleague, or even the team) to obtain guidance about what can and cannot be discussed. Providers' emotions, reactions, and behavior will be essential to discuss with the team; particular details about the client's death may need to be discussed only with the carrier or one's attorney. The team agreement in Chapter 2 is designed to establish team information as confidential; however, we know of no precedent establishing this, and confidential material may still be requested in certain legal situations. The malpractice carrier can provide guidance for these issues.

- The team may also need to help the provider follow the recommendations of the malpractice carrier, if the provider is not in wise mind. The team can help them to practice wise mind exercises, use crisis survival strategies, and otherwise help to manage intense emotion. The team can also remind the provider that by implementing an evidence-based treatment that incorporates regular, effective risk assessments and a team, they not only have provided the best treatment possible, but these strategies can offer some protection from a liability standpoint. Following the DBT manual and documenting one has done so can help establish that the provider has done their best to provide effective responses to crisis situations. These interventions can help calm the provider so they can respond most effectively to consultation.

• Most importantly, remember that litigation regarding a suicide is rare, and there is help available. Grieving the loss of a client is difficult enough without adding the concern of legal difficulties. Therapy, legal consultation, and other assistance may be needed to navigate such a challenging situation.

• After some time has passed and emotions have calmed somewhat, the DBT team can facilitate a review of the client's chart. (Seek consultation from the malpractice carrier regarding how to do so.) The primary therapist and/or team leader can check the client's chart notes to determine if all notes are complete and signed, risk assessments are in place, and there is evidence the provider was tracking and treating suicide risk. In the event that there are notes missing, or anything in the chart that increases concerns, this can be a very distressing discovery! Do not alter the medical record; instead, the primary therapist or team leader can obtain consultation from the malpractice carrier. The malpractice carrier will offer advice and instructions. In some cases, the malpractice carrier may also assign an attorney to assist; the relevant team members can ask for support from the team leader or other members to navigate these conversations, particularly if emotions are high (while again, following advice regarding keeping certain details of the death in confidence, if recommended to do so by the malpractice carrier).

Supporting Each Other

After the death of a client, the team's main job is to support each other: this includes the primary therapist, skills trainers, other team members who had contact with the client, as well as members who had never met the client. This may include administrative staff who work with the team as well. Team members may have a variety of reactions to the suicide, including anger, grief, shame, fear, relief, numbness, a loss of confidence, and/or a loss of motivation to provide DBT or to treat difficult clients (for more information about provider responses to client suicides, see, e.g., Hendin, Lipschitz, Maltsberger, Haas, & Wynecoop, 2000; Ruskin, Safinosky, Bagby, Dickens, & Sousa, 2004; Draper, Kolves, DeLeo, &

Snowdon, 2014; and Gulfi, Castelli Dransart, Heeb, & Gutjahr, 2015). Some may even experience acute stress disorder or PTSD (Ruskin et al., 2004). Some team members may feel relief or report no distress at all. All of these reactions are normative.

The team should directly assess how each member is doing, rather than assume they are "fine." Overtly ask about emotions, thoughts including self-blame, urges, and what resources they have to deal with their own reactions. The team can ask about changes in behavior or attitude toward other clients and DBT more broadly, including more avoidance of discussing suicide, urges to hospitalize clients, irritability toward clients, rumination, and desire to quit providing DBT or to change careers. It is helpful to directly ask every member of the team about these experiences. While it is useful to obtain consultation with the malpractice carrier or legal representative before discussing in team a particular team member's culpability, it is perfectly acceptable and important to discuss emotions, thoughts, and other reactions, and essential to obtain intensive support from the team.

Certain team members may be more likely to experience strong reactions such as guilt, doubt, and self-blame. For example, the primary therapist may have a more intense reaction, as the "hub of the wheel" in the treatment who created the treatment plan and monitored risk. Alternatively, some team members will say they do not need anything; experience has taught us that even in those cases, it is important to assess and offer support repeatedly; the need for support may develop over time, as emotions and events evolve. In a survey conducted with Swiss mental health and social professionals, providers who reported insufficient support also reported experiencing greater impact from the suicide (Castelli, Dransart, Heeb, Gulfi, & Gutjahr, 2015), so this support is essential.

Due to the nature of the role, the team may neglect to assess the needs of the team leader, who may also be vulnerable to intense reactions after a suicide. The team leader's reaction may be different from others on the team. As the leader of the team and the one with oversight of the DBT program, the team leader may feel a greater sense of responsibility for the suicide and be especially prone to guilt, anxiety, and self-invalidating thoughts. The leader may feel torn between several demands, including managing the needs of the primary therapist, the team, the client's family, and the agency, and may as a result neglect their own needs. There may be a sense of being out of control or anger if the leader feels unsupported by the agency, or believes a teammate did not follow a protocol. It is important for the team to assess the needs of the team leader, and for the leader to seek support.

Primary forms of support may include a lot of validation, along with guidance if a team member is using ineffective strategies to cope, or needs instructions for how to proceed. Teammates can remind each other that the entire team is treating the client, and that none of them is alone in this experience; this is a community of therapists. The team can also offer inspiration and motivation. Suicidal individuals have an extremely difficult time finding effective care, and the fact that the team is willing to provide care to those individuals is profound and meaningful, even if it carries with it the risk of suicide. To drop the team's risk of suicide to zero would mean not offering the treatment to those for whom it was designed: those with multiple, chronic problems and high suicide risk. Remembering why team members chose to learn this treatment can help combat hopelessness and doubts that may arise after a client's death.

After the initial discussion regarding the suicide, the team may also benefit from additional, more formal meeting(s) or a retreat to address the team's reaction. The quicker such a meeting can be scheduled, the better, but it does not need to be within days of receiving the news of a client's suicide. The team leader and other members can generate activities for these meetings, including talking, free-writing, and conducting exercises. For example, after a suicide in our (JS) team, we held a retreat that was scheduled for 3 hours. With input from team members, we did the following:

- We ate soothing food.
- We met in an environment outside of work (a team member's living room).
- Each person shared with the group how they were feeling about the suicide, other clients, and more generally. We discussed changes in team members' behavior, such as looking up information about the death online, having urges to stop working with other high-risk clients, and recommending other clients be hospitalized more frequently than usual. The team validated these responses extensively.
- The team leader reminded the team that they were doing profound work. They were helping those who struggled to find help elsewhere, because of the high suicide risk.
- The team leader reminded the team that they were not in the business of controlling clients' behavior. They teach new ways to respond

to distress, but they cannot and do not want to control clients' every move. This leaves room for suicide to occur, and such risk is part of implementing DBT. No one knows how to completely prevent suicide; the team can only offer their best strategies to help clients build lives that are experienced as worth living.

● We completed the Cope Ahead exercise (pp. 163–165): We focused on each member's worst fear as a result of this suicide, and used imaginal rehearsal to practice coping. Each member shared with the team.

● We discussed that this suicide presented each of them with a fork in the road. This could either make one feel hopeless and demoralized or it could galvanize them, and that one could influence the impact the suicide would have. Each member responded to the question, "Why do we do this work?" Each member came up with specific reasons, including clients who experienced significant success with DBT, and other clients who still need help. This was similar to the Pros and Cons exercise above; it helped remind each other that there are strong reasons to continue doing this work, even in the most painful moments.

The team may also need to be vigilant for signs that the distress the team member is experiencing is interfering with other clients' treatment. A provider may become more reactive to clients' mention of suicide, or become emotional in sessions in a way that is not helpful. There may be more anxiety or anger with other clients. The urge to hospitalize clients may increase dramatically, as well as efforts to control client behavior; a team member may also lose faith that the treatment is effective. The team must discuss the potential for these changes, and, if there are concerns, watch or listen to recordings of certain sessions. It is important to note that having these reactions is common, and not a sign that a provider should stop work or cannot recover; it is simply a sign that more assistance may be needed. The team can use all of the DBT assessment and intervention strategies to help alleviate these problems. At times, a team member's needs may be beyond what the team can manage; in these cases the team may recommend that a team member attend individual therapy in addition to receiving support in the team. It will also be important to note that this need for support may go on much longer than some may expect, and the team may need to be vigilant for the team member's needs for an extended period of time. A formal system for checking in may be useful, such as having teammates contact the distressed team member regularly with scheduled calls.

Monitoring Team Functioning

A client suicide may, in some cases, lead to more tense or avoidant team interactions. A team member may not feel supported enough, or interpret the team's reactions as blaming. A team member may stop speaking in team for a period of time, due to shame, fear, or anger. Alternatively, the team may believe a certain member did not intervene sufficiently before the suicide, and experience emotion and urges regarding that individual. Typically, teams will be warm and supportive and offer help to the affected team members, but on occasion teams will struggle in these extremely difficult circumstances. Using the strategies described in this book (e.g., validating extensively, referring to the team agreements, assessing carefully, problem solving) will be useful. Most importantly, remaining aware that the team may go through a period of tension, and that emotions are higher than usual but will likely return to normal at some point, can help ground the team and heighten skills use for this period of time.

Interacting with the Family

Certain team members and the team at large may know the family of the client well, or may have had no contact with them at all. The family may not have been aware that the individual was in treatment. In most cases, contacting the family is recommended, and is viewed as important and helpful, even if the family is distressed and even angry at the primary therapist or team. While the team may not be directly involved in the communications with the family, this topic is very relevant to the DBT team, because the team is a community of therapists treating the client. At a minimum, the primary therapist and team leader should be communicating regularly about these decisions; the entire team can offer input and guidance as well.

There are certain factors for the team to consider when contacting the family. None of these recommendations constitute legal advice; typically these situations are quite complex and at times may require consultation from an expert such as one's malpractice carrier or legal counsel. We can, however, highlight issues that may be relevant to the DBT team, and suggest guidance and resources such that these situations are navigated effectively.

As we have previously mentioned, the first step after a suicide, prior to contacting the family, is to contact one's malpractice carrier or legal counsel. This is a time to obtain advice about communicating with the family and the relevant variables to consider. In most cases, it will be recommended that the provider contacts the family. In these interactions, it is important to be compassionate, genuine, and open. Family members are often comforted and moved by such gestures. If the provider is closed up, cool, or defensive, or avoids the family altogether, whether out of fear or grief or other reactions, the family may misinterpret this as disinterest, detachment, or defensiveness. Ideally, the provider can try to convey, in a very genuine style, their own grief and concern for the family's well-being. The provider may need the team's help (e.g., emotion regulation and/or role playing) to prepare for this contact, particularly if they are in high distress. In situations where a team member is too upset to talk calmly to the family right away, the team leader or another teammate can help them make the call, or even contact the family first if needed.

Confidentiality will be important to consider, as it continues beyond the death of a client (although there are a few exceptions to this; see the U.S. Department of Health and Human Services [2013], Health Information of Deceased Individual, retrieved from *www.hhs.gov/hipaa/for-professionals/privacy/guidance/health-information-of-deceased-individuals/index.html*). It is important to remember the family may not have known the client was in therapy, and contacting the family in some cases may itself violate confidentiality.

If the family wishes to obtain more information from the team or the client's records, this information cannot be shared with the family unless/until they become or obtain permission from a "personal representative" (e.g., executor) of the client. Being open with the family regarding the reasons for withholding information will be essential to avoid misunderstandings; the provider might explain, "I'm so sorry I can't say more; I know this information would help you process what has happened. I still have to maintain his confidentiality, even though I know that's hard for you. Only the personal representative can give me permission to share more." Even with such permission, the family may also wish to consider the client's wishes; the provider might say, "It is worth thinking about whether he would have wanted his family to see his therapy notes; that decision is up to you, but something to consider." The provider may also describe the team's procedures for assessing and monitoring risk to the family, which may be comforting to the family without disclosing personal details pertaining to the client. A delicate balance is struck between protecting the client's privacy and attending to the family's grief, all while the team member is regulating their own emotions. This is not easy in the wake of a suicide, and the team member may need the team's help to communicate with the family.

Because the client was being treated by the entire team, the entire team may wish to express condolences to the family. The family may not wish to have personal contact with each member of the team but the team can show support with a card or flowers, for example. Members of the team, and in particular the primary therapist, skills trainers, and program leader may also wish to attend the funeral/memorial service. Families will vary on whether they wish to keep the services small, or want support from a large number of people. The primary therapist or team leader can be the liaison for such communication to avoid overwhelming the family.

See Sung (2016a, 2016b) for more guidance regarding contacting family members.

Informing Other Clients

If the deceased client was attending a skills group, or otherwise interacted with other clients, it will be important to inform other clients of the death. This will require the entire team to work together to manage the potential increase in suicide risk for other clients. Some of the clients may be in close contact with each other, so it will be important to synchronize the notifications if at all possible, such that clients hear it first from their own provider and not from another client. The team can agree on the amount of information to be disclosed and the timing. We recommend these notifications occur prior to the next skills group, so that the information is delivered individually before it is brought up in a group setting.

Team members must be careful to acknowledge clients' sadness, fear, and other reactions that occur, helping clients skillfully experience any emotion that may arise. Just like team members, clients may have a wide range of emotions, including anger and numbness. Their reactions can be normalized and validated. At the same time, providers will need to be careful not to glorify the suicide (e.g., extensively praising the client who died, or emphasizing that they are in a much better, more peaceful place). In the skills group, the skills leaders can spend a portion of the time acknowledging the situation, modeling effective expression of emotion, and offering validation and skills; returning to the skills curriculum after a period of time may be distressing to clients, but will be important to avoid reinforcing suicide as a solution. The skills leaders may repeat this process in the subsequent 1–2 skills groups by spending 15 minutes on skills pertaining to coping with the suicide and then returning to the normal curriculum.

Team members will also need to monitor for high suicide risk, and stay in close contact with those who may need extra coaching or support. Clients may interpret the death to mean DBT doesn't work. All members of the team can emphasize that this client is different from the deceased client (e.g., "She did not stay in treatment long enough for it to work" or "He gave up and you haven't,") and coach them in using skills to tolerate the distress of the news.

All of this is particularly difficult, given that providers will be experiencing their own intense emotions while managing these clients' reactions and risk. If team members are highly emotional themselves, they may need help from the team to regulate their own emotions sufficiently to be helpful to clients. For example, if a client blames a team member for the suicide, or becomes silent and will not answer questions or respond to validation, that provider may become highly distressed given their intense vulnerability. Team members will need to communicate frequently during this period, to be sure clients are attended to, and team members are regulated enough to do so. Team members can help each other by jumping in with each other's clients if needed, offering Crisis Survival and Emotion Regulation skills, validation, and any other interventions that will help the clients and providers get through a very challenging time. And once again, obtaining consultation within and outside of team is always helpful after a suicide.

Finding Meaning

Given how difficult a client suicide is to deal with and recover from, it may be important to find meaning in the experience. The skill of Finding Meaning, from the IMPROVE skill (Linehan, 2015a, 2015b), refers to finding some element of purpose, meaning, or benefit from a highly distressing event. It is important to note that this is a dialectical skill—in other words, this skill does not suggest one moves from one pole ("This is bad") to the other pole ("This is good, I shouldn't feel bad about this"), but to hold both poles true at once. In other words, this suicide causes tremendous sadness, anger, and pain, *and* some meaning can be found in it.

One of the best ways to find meaning in a client suicide is to learn from the experience, and improve services for other current and potential clients. If the team can learn from the action of one client, future suicides or other crises may be prevented. This process could be conducted through a discussion or exercise in team, or can be more detailed, such as a formal review of clinic policies. Team members can ask, "Is there something here that could benefit our clients?" This question is not asked in a manner that seeks to blame or judge, but from a truly curious standpoint. The team could do this together, or the primary therapist could engage in this process with a teammate or team leader, and any conclusions can be shared with the entire team. Such findings may also lead to changes in policies, procedures, and treatment forms.

For example, after a suicide, one DBT provider we worked with reviewed everything that had happened in the last few sessions, including discussions, interventions, risk assessments, and session notes. She concluded that while she followed all of the procedures effectively, the client died by suicide anyway. This led to two interventions: first, the team completed an exercise focused on radically accepting that all of the strategies they had may still be insufficient at times. It was helpful for the team to discuss that there was no foolproof way to prevent suicide, and that this client population was already at elevated risk for death from suicide. They discussed how each team member did the very best they could with every client, this effort was met with success most of the time, *and* most DBT providers will be affected by a client suicide at some point. This exercise was done in the hopes of helping team members decrease their fear and remain in wise mind after a suicide. The team also brainstormed changes in procedures, and decided to add a "crisis card" form for clients to keep in their wallets, with skills and phone numbers to be used in a crisis.

Another way to find meaning is to complete the Pros and Cons skill (Linehan, 2015a, 2015b), focused on the pros and cons of treating suicidal clients. This exercise can help the team to remember that even in the most painful moments, when one is most fearful or saddened or angered by a client's life-threatening actions, there are reasons why we do this work. Teams can complete the worksheet individually, then have a team discussion of why this work remains so meaningful and valuable. Pros of treating these clients can include one's values, particular clients who have benefitted in the past or who are benefitting currently from treatment, future clients one will help, a sense of satisfaction and contribution, and so on. Cons of seeing these clients might include one's emotions regarding suicide, fear of liability, and other consequences experienced or imagined. Pros of avoidance might include less fear or worry, and escape from the current difficult situation; cons of avoidance might be feeling one is not fulfilling one's purpose. Emphasizing the pros of treating these clients and the cons of avoiding them can help increase team members' motivation, even when stress is high. This exercise may help everyone in the team reconnect with the deep meaning to be found in providing DBT. Acknowledging the difficulties treating suicidal clients, and remembering all the reasons we do this work anyway, can both build motivation and help identify those who are struggling, so the team can move in and help.

Conclusion

There are many steps team members may wish to take with respect to managing client suicide risk, including taking care of oneself, obtaining outside consultation, seeking training to recognize and manage risk, and attending therapy. This chapter focuses solely on the importance of the DBT team when coping with suicide crisis. The team can provide support; facilitate even more effective therapeutic interventions before, during, and after a suicide crisis; and help each team member act effectively for their own, the clients', and the team's benefit.

IDEAS FOR PRACTICE

- Complete one or more exercises regarding client suicide risk, from this chapter or elsewhere, either as a team or individually.
- Attend a training focused on suicide assessment and/or management. Share what you learn with your team.
- Have a team discussion about the meaning of this work. Ask yourself:
  - What about this work brings me meaning, personally?
  - Why did I pursue learning DBT in the first place?
  - Why have I continued even when the work was very difficult?

- What about this work brings meaning to us as a community?
- Think of a client who benefitted from DBT. Where would that person be if I had not provided DBT?
- Think of a current client. What would happen to them if I burned out and kept treating them but was too frustrated or too frightened to provide effective care?

■ Have a team discussion about what happens when providers try to control their clients.

■ Write out, then discuss, what obstacles each team member may face in dealing with high-risk situations. How do you typically respond when experiencing intense fear, shame, or other emotions that could arise when working with high-risk clients? How might the team be helpful in those situations? Brainstorm how each team member can best provide and receive help effectively before, during, and after a suicide crisis.

Starting a DBT Team

B efore a team can run successfully, multiple decisions must be made regarding how to start. The goal will always be to maximize adherence to the treatment manual, as discussed previously. We have found it works well to make mindful decisions regarding the structure and agreements for the team, and, as we have discussed throughout this book, there are many ways to do this. For example, a large team or a team with fewer experienced DBT clinicians may require greater structure; a small team with highly experienced clinicians may need very little. Many teams will find they need to reorganize and revise their structure as their teams develop. This chapter describes strategies for starting a DBT team and bringing on new team members.

Below is a list of the common steps teams typically face as they start. These steps fall into two general categories: program and membership. Some of these steps will be less relevant depending on the circumstance; remember the idea is not to rigidly follow these suggestions, but instead to use this list to guide and support team members' capability and motivation.

Programmatic Processes

1. Create a training plan.

2. Decide which clients will and will not be treated by the team.

3. Define which aspects of the treatment will be provided/adapted.

4. Determine when, where, and how long the team will meet.

Membership Processes

1. Decide on the size of the team.

2. Select new team members.

3. Have an orientation and commitment discussion with potential members.

4. Assign team roles.

Programmatic Processes
Creating a Training Plan

We have met many individuals who are highly motivated to start a DBT team, but they do not have sufficient expertise to know how to provide effective DBT. This is not a reason to slow down! The team can simply make obtaining training their first goal. Reading the DBT manuals, attending trainings, and seeking consultation will all likely be useful in expanding knowledge and expertise. The team may also consider recruiting a more experienced DBT provider to join and facilitate the launch of the new team. Some teams may begin team meetings prior to seeing clients, and the first team meetings will focus on training, marketing, and other tasks aimed at starting a program. In other teams, team members will already have caseloads when they join together to form a team. We typically recommend teams start small, seeing just a few DBT clients in the beginning, paying as much attention to adherence as possible. This seems to be a more effective way to learn the treatment and run the team effectively, rather than starting with many clients and less focus on closely following the manual. Each team will have its unique circumstances and can choose its own path, obtaining consultation as needed.

Deciding Which Clients Will and Will Not Be Treated by the Team

There is flexibility in whom the team treats; what is important is that the team has an established scope of services for its members, and a clear understanding of which clients will be treated and discussed by the team. These decisions should be based on research data, team members' training and experience, and treatment setting. Such variables include age range, diagnoses, presenting problems, and any exclusion criteria such as active psychosis, cognitive ability, or other factors. The team does not need to have a very narrow range of services; for example, not everyone needs to treat just BPD or just eating disorders, and different members may have different criteria (e.g., only some team members will work with teens). While there are no rules about whom the team may treat or exclude, clear inclusion criteria will allow the team to exclude individuals who do not fit the established model. For example, in DBT, the team should only treat those clients for whom there are data suggesting DBT may be helpful. If the team decides to make an exception to this, team members should mindfully and thoughtfully make this decision, inform the client, and monitor the effectiveness of the intervention. The DBT team will not treat clients who are receiving interventions such as supportive "talk therapy" and psychodynamic therapy. These clients will have a non-DBT, nonbehavioral conceptualization and remain off the DBT team. The team will also exclude those clients for whom research suggests there is a more effective treatment than that provided by the team (e.g., a DBT team would not treat someone who has panic disorder with no other diagnoses; this case would likely do best with CBT for panic disorder, and therefore it would not be discussed in team). It is also important for the providers in the team to work within their area of competence. Setting inclusion and exclusion criteria can provide a helpful structure for these decisions. Teams will need to have a system for assessing clients to determine whether they will be treated by the team, and a person who manages this system (often the team leader). For example, our (JS) team has one individual who speaks to all potential clients by phone and asks screening questions about the areas of dysregulation (emotional dysregulation, interpersonal dysregulation, behavioral dysregulation, cognitive dysregulation, and dysregulation of the sense of self; Linehan, 1993). This helps begin the process of determining who will be a good fit for the team; for those the brief screen identifies as possible candidates for DBT, the screen is followed by a careful diagnostic interview. The team leader establishes the system and sets the criteria for inclusion and exclusion. Each team will benefit from setting criteria and identifying the individual(s) who will make such decisions.

Defining Which Aspects of the Treatment Will Be Provided or Adapted

As will be discussed below, it is essential that all DBT team members agree to provide DBT, and agree upon which components of DBT will be included in treatment. Teams may opt to provide comprehensive DBT in the traditional manner, or they may choose to offer certain components (e.g., team and skills training), or offer the functions of DBT in an atypical manner (e.g., inpatient settings). These choices should be made based on available data and from a single theoretical approach, strategically rather than in a reactive manner. What is essential here is that the team have a clear, precise approach to clients; it can detract from consultation if team members speak different languages (i.e., have differing theoretical perspectives), or have different approaches to understanding, conceptualizing, and treating particular behaviors. (As a side note, it is also important to communicate clearly to clients when a team decides not to provide comprehensive DBT, such that they are not led to believe they have received a comprehensive treatment when they have not.)

Teams may also provide other CBT interventions within the DBT structure (e.g., within DBT one might implement many additional evidence-based treatments for problems such as anxiety, depression, or sleep disorders; this decision will be based on the case conceptualization and what the data suggest are most effective and relevant for clients' particular problems). These are not considered adaptations to DBT; other evidence-based treatments are often incorporated into DBT when treating problems that severely interfere with a client's quality of life.

Determining When, Where, and How Long the Team Will Meet

As discussed in Chapter 1, DBT team members are expected to treat DBT team time just as they would a therapy session, meaning they attend regularly and do not double-book, whenever possible. Therefore, decisions about team logistics should set up conditions so all members can attend regularly. Team logistics typically include:

- What time?
- Where?
- How long?
- How often?

What Time?

Since team members are asked to consider team as important as any therapy session, team members will be expected to attend the *entire* meeting. Therefore, the time should not be set such that one or more members must miss a portion of team regularly. If administration does not provide time for a team meeting, members can work to convince the administration of the importance of team (including such reasons as decreasing liability by including an essential component of an evidence-based treatment, providing better care, and addressing provider burnout, all of which may be very important to administration; this topic is discussed more in Chapter 3), or arrange the team meeting on their own time, such as during the lunch hour (which may actually add to burnout; arranging team time on members' own time must be within their limits to work effectively). Once the time is set, all providers will establish their schedules around this meeting, so maintaining its stability is very helpful. If a team member cannot attend regularly, they may need to exit the team until regular attendance becomes possible.

Where?

The team will ideally meet in person; team members may also meet via video conferencing or phone, if necessary. The focus of the team is to treat the providers rather than the clients; therefore, it is not necessary that the providers are in the same agency or treat the same clients. Team members can discuss the travel or technology necessary to attend the meeting. In rural settings, providers may live at great distance from one another yet have a fully functioning DBT team. (Be certain to provide informed consent regarding team membership to each client, and carefully protect clients' identities if team members are not at the same agency. For example, obtain releases to discuss cases with colleagues and use a HIPAA-compliant video conferencing service if the team is conducted via video conference.) Because team members provide therapy for the therapist, meeting in person is likely most effective; however, it is not required. Once again, team members can choose the set-up that best facilitates their capability and motivation, based upon their own unique circumstances.

Teams also need to choose a room or setting for their meetings. There is plenty of flexibility with the physical space, as long as the size

of the room (large enough to accommodate all members) and the privacy of the room (members can feel comfortable discussing their clients
and themselves without being overheard) are sufficient. Team members
may prefer a conference table with a whiteboard and projector so all
members can view case formulations and session videos during team.

How Long?

The length of the team will vary based on the number of members, the
number of clients carried in a team, and other variables. At a minimum,
we have found that 1 hour is needed, even when teams are as small as
two to three members. Larger teams, such as those with eight members,
may need 2 hours to get through their agendas successfully. Teams can
weigh the pros and cons and choose the length of time based on the
team's needs.

How Often?

Teams should meet regularly, not on an as-needed basis. We recommend
meeting once per week for outpatient care; inpatient settings may require
more frequent, even daily, contact.

Membership Processes
Deciding on the Size of the Team

DBT teams consist of at least two people. Most teams seem to thrive
with three to eight members. In our experience, at a certain size teams
have more difficulty meeting the needs of the members. Teams of over
12 members may become too large; at that size, the team may need to
develop strategies for managing the size of the team, or divide into two
teams. We both have been on large teams that have worked well, and
large teams that lost their effectiveness due to their size. Very small
teams may decide they are too small, as well; with only two members, for
example, it may be difficult to remain dialectical. The experience of team
members, size of caseloads, and other variables may influence this decision. Teams can monitor the effectiveness of the meetings and determine
what size is the best for them.

Selecting New Team Members

We have provided consultation to many teams regarding the selection of team members. First and foremost, teams will benefit from mindfully generating a list of team agreements based on those described in Chapter 1, orienting interested individuals in a direct and open manner, and inviting in only those who are fully committed to those agreements. In other words, we are rather choosy about who joins our teams! We have seen a variety of difficulties arise regarding team membership, and have found that when teams are thoughtful about team culture and agreements, they are able to minimize problems. In addition to those agreements, we have provided a list below that suggests additional discussion topics and elements to consider.

Voluntary Membership

As we have discussed previously, it is important that DBT team members join voluntarily, with a clear understanding of what will be asked of them. While many of the other guidelines suggested here are quite flexible, voluntary membership is an essential ingredient of an effective team. Part of the commitment phase of joining a team includes an orientation to the team, how it functions, and the expectations for members. Even in agencies where all staff are expected to be on a DBT team, it will help the team culture significantly if all members commit to the team by choice. In cases where DBT team is a requirement of employment, this commitment phase can be completed during the job interview process (this is discussed further, below, with respect to commitment strategies). It is important to accept members who commit fully to the team's agreements, and to turn away those who are not interested in following those agreements (e.g., those who commit to some but not all agreements, or give a vague or "wishy-washy" commitment). For the team to be successful, all members will need to join voluntarily, and fully agree to the principles and agreements of the DBT team.

Willingness to Be Vulnerable

As we discussed in Chapter 1, it is essential to focus on the willingness to be vulnerable when selecting new team members. In our experience, teams do not work well if one or some members do not show vulnerability within the team meeting. In order for therapy for the therapist to be successful, each team member must be willing to engage in behaviors that enhance vulnerability, including sharing mistakes and uncertainty, skillfully allowing one's own emotion to arise in team, grappling with others' emotion in team meetings, and being open to connection with and feedback from teammates. This openness in team is central to the process of therapy for the therapist, and essential for the DBT team to run effectively.

Clinical responsibility is a key element of establishing a culture of vulnerability in DBT team. When each individual has some type of client contact, differences in power and status are more likely to be navigated successfully. If an individual in team does not have or speak about clinical responsibility (e.g., one member attends in a supervisory role but does not discuss their own clinical work, or is a peer but does not see any clients, and therefore can provide suggestions to others but never receives any feedback), it can significantly affect the team's ability to provide therapy for the therapist. When one member is not vulnerable in this way, other team members may hide mistakes, feel too embarrassed to share their struggles, or feel resentful that individuals oversimplify the ease of solving a problem when they do not have firsthand knowledge of the difficulty of the situation.

It is often unavoidable to have people of different hierarchical positions on the team (e.g., supervisor and supervisee, boss and employee, administrator and staff). While this can create fundamental differences in the level of vulnerability, this situation also has its benefits. For example, having administrators on the team may make them better able to support the team, and having supervisors on the team will likely enhance their ability to supervise. When individuals with relatively more power model fallibility, it helps to set the tone and will increase the likelihood that other members will also do so. If individuals in higher power positions (e.g., administrators) are to remain on the team, it is important for them to have a clinical role and responsibility of some kind (i.e., not just saying hello to clients in the milieu). All team members need to be "down in the trenches" together in order to establish the culture necessary for therapy for the therapist. Having each member experience at firsthand the practical as well as emotional challenges of providing DBT will place members on a more equal playing field.

Professional Qualifications

Team members must decide which professions or areas of specialization will join the team. There are no a priori restrictions on the type of degree members of the team must have. Sufficient education, training, supervision, and license (or licensed supervisor) for their particular role is essential, but this will look different across teams. In many settings, multiple providers interact with DBT clients. Not all of these providers will join the DBT team; teams will vary widely in terms of the number of different professions on the team. This does not always need to be decided a priori, and teams may remain flexible about which providers participate in team.

At a minimum, all members, regardless of profession, can be considered for membership on the team if they follow the team agreements, including holding clinical responsibility for DBT clients, and provide interventions within the DBT model. It is also important for team members to have some knowledge of the particular problems or diagnoses treated by the team. This is important because the team is treating each client as a community, not as a set of individual providers, and it will be difficult for team members to monitor fidelity to the treatment manual, to support each other sufficiently, and to challenge each other if the team members do not know anything about the particular problem area. For example, if the team uses DBT primarily to treat clients presenting with eating disorders, the team members will benefit from having at least some expertise in eating disorders as well as DBT, in order to be effective consultants for each other. Other teams may simply require expertise in DBT; they may treat a variety of DBT clients, and aside from a shared understanding of DBT, each member has a niche or area of specialization that is not shared by other members. Teams or agencies may also require DBT certification (or progress toward certification) as a condition of membership.

Provider Roles with Clients

We have had a variety of roles in our teams over the years. We have concluded that only two are absolutely essential to the functioning of the team (individual therapist and skills trainer), and others can be optional depending on the team's needs.

There may be situations in which the individual therapist and skills trainers will be on different teams. There are definite cons to this approach, but in some circumstances the pros may outweigh those cons. Teams can discuss the dialectic inherent in this situation and come to the best arrangement for the clients and the providers. For example, in agencies where the number of DBT providers requires two separate teams, a client may end up seeing an individual therapist who attends one team and skills trainers who attend another. Logistically, this situation may be impossible to avoid in larger programs, or in situations where private practitioners with independent practices join with colleagues for their DBT team.

Additional provider roles may also attend team (and in our view, as long as the team does not get too large, the more that can attend, the better!):

- Pharmacotherapists
- Case managers
- Milieu coaches
- Physicians
- Nurses
- Line staff
- Teachers
- Family therapists
- Recreational therapists

Any of these individuals may be on the team, in which case they fulfill the DBT team agreements and provide their interventions within the DBT model.

Those providers who do not operate within DBT principles, but have contact with the client, remain off the team and are considered "ancillary." This means that the provider is not on the team and is not expected to follow DBT principles. In such cases, the client can work to ensure that the ancillary provider is not working against their DBT treatment using the individual therapist as a consultant in this process (see "Consultation to the Patient"; Linehan, 1993); the DBT provider can also engage in environmental interventions when useful.

Attending Multiple DBT Teams

In a non-DBT team, there are no issues with attending two teams, because the focus is only on the clients in each team. However, in a DBT team, the focus is on the team member, not the client, meaning that attending two teams could be likened to a client working with two therapists. This does not mean one cannot attend two teams; however, we recommend that this is only done rarely and with great care.

Receiving therapy from two teams can be challenging for the provider. We have both attended two teams when on research or training teams, in addition to our ongoing team. We both noticed it was more difficult to be vulnerable and receive therapy in the team that met later in the week because we had received consultation in the first team earlier in the week. Our second teams noticed we were less engaged.

In situations where attending two teams becomes a necessity, mindful engagement in both teams is needed. First, it's important that all involved parties are aware of those who are attending two teams. The team may need to discuss and determine whether the team can tolerate members attending more than one team simultaneously and identify how to best handle any difficulties. One helpful strategy can be for the provider to clearly distinguish which clients are associated with which team, and then bring up obstacles to treating those clients in that particular team. If the provider is experiencing a life situation that is impeding treatment for clients in both teams, the topic can be discussed in both teams. Individuals struggling with being on two teams can benefit from discussing this dilemma in team, to obtain help with fully engaging in both teams. The team can also remain aware of the potential difficulties; this presents an opportunity for a dialectical conversation regarding the team member's capability and motivation. Attending two teams is possible with care but may not be the ideal choice for some individuals.

Handling Multiple Roles within the Team

Some team members may have additional relationship roles with each other, which can present dialectical challenges within the team. In addition to supervisor/supervisee roles, for example, team members may be close friends or even romantic partners. To forbid such relationships would be impractical and also nondialectical. Instead, we suggest that teams assess and determine how to manage such roles. There may be times where having business partners or romantic partners on the same team enhances team functioning, and times when such dual roles could create difficulties on the team. Such situations are opportunities for the team to present both poles and come to a synthesis, rather than having a "rule" about how to manage multiple roles.

Having an Orientation and Commitment Discussion with Potential Members

Regardless of the process by which the team is built, a clear orientation and commitment process is needed. In this process, each new member agrees to the team agreements, which ensures that each member joining the team wishes to function within this type of team, and provides an opportunity to depart prior to joining if it is not a good match. Orienting and obtaining commitment can also help to highlight areas where the team may need to troubleshoot potential problems with maintaining the team culture (remembering that the team does not ask for perfection; instead, the team focuses on a desire to aspire to the team agreements, even if certain skills are not yet fully developed). The team member(s) conducting this session will likely be more effective if they are neutral and curious about whether the potential member is interested in making a commitment to the DBT team, rather than attempting to convince the individual to join. The orientation and commitment session can entail a genuine, frank discussion about the individual's desire to join the team and abide by the structure and culture set out by the team.

Obviously, this orientation and commitment session should be conducted before an individual joins the team. Team leaders do not need to readily accept every individual who volunteers to join. While in most settings it can be assumed that the individual is motivated to join the team based on the decision to approach the team, in other settings the process may be less voluntary (e.g., an agency begins using DBT and all existing employees are required to join a DBT team). A potential member may be very eager but not well informed as to what the team requires as well.

This process often occurs as a conversation between a new member and an existing team member. Potential team members may have this discussion with the team leader, a team member, or in some cases the entire team. Conducting an orientation and commitment session in front of a large team can feel overwhelming or even coercive, and may reduce the chances of a genuine commitment; meeting with the potential member individually or with a small number of team members is likely more effective when teams have more than three or four members.

In some settings, team members may find it helpful to commit to a certain period of time (e.g., 1 year), just as clients in DBT do, with an assessment and recommitment session at the end of that time period. The commitment period should be long enough to provide continuity to the team and sufficient time to provide DBT to one's clients. (For example, if one is an individual DBT therapist, 1 year will likely be the minimum commitment period for the team; those providing skills training or other modes of treatment may have a different required length of commitment such as 6 months; the team may wish to require a longer commitment to avoid repeated transitions in team.)

The orientation and commitment process may look very different in different teams. Some teams may prefer to have a highly structured process for each incoming team member; other teams may be very flexible and tailor the commitment process to the individual joining the team. The process may take very little time, if the individual has been on a DBT team before, or may require more time and detail if the individual is not aware of the many differences between a DBT team and a more traditional consultation team. It should be emphasized to the potential member that a DBT team is best viewed as therapy for the therapist, in which team members are implementing DBT with each other in order to maintain provider capability and motivation. Below is a list of specific orientation topics that are typically covered in the orientation and commitment meeting.

- The function of the DBT team (fidelity; capability and motivation of team members).
- Whom will be treated by the DBT team and how (e.g., client population, components of treatment provided, other necessary areas of expertise or training).
- When the team meets, for how long, and any other relevant team information.
- How the team time is spent (i.e., the agenda, providing therapy for the therapist).

- The roles in the DBT team.
- The culture of the team.
  - DBT team agreements
  - DBT assumptions about clients and therapy

The exact content of this orientation will be informed by the team's unique needs.

Discussion of DBT Team Agreements

The culture of the team requires careful attention during the orientation and commitment process, particularly if this potential member has not been on a DBT team before. DBT team agreements were discussed in more detail in Chapter 1, and are only listed here.

Core DBT Team Agreements

1. Dialectical Agreement.
2. Consultation-to-the-Client Agreement.
3. Consistency Agreement.
4. Observing-Limits Agreement.
5. Phenomenological Empathy Agreement.
6. Fallibility Agreement.

To these six core DBT team agreements, we have added additional agreements that most teams find helpful. This is the expanded list of DBT team agreements (see Chapter 1), which includes:

7. Consider oneself part of a community of therapists treating a community of clients.
8. Provide "therapy for the therapist."
9. Provide DBT.
10. Conceptualize clients' and each other's behavior from a behavioral perspective.
11. Treat team meetings as importantly as any other therapy session.
12. Be available to fulfill the role for which one joined the team.

13. Be willing to call out the "elephant in the room" when others do not.

14. Remain one-mindful in team.

15. Assess sufficiently before offering solutions.

16. Strive to follow the assumptions about clients and therapy.

17. Follow team policy regarding providing coverage for each other, missing team, and missing appointments with clients.

18. Continue focusing on all of the above, even when feeling burned out, frustrated, tired, overworked, underappreciated, hopeless, ineffective, etc.

There is a dialectic within these team agreements: on the one hand, it is extremely helpful to obtain a commitment from a new team member to adhere to these agreements; they help to maintain the culture of the team and prevent team problems as time progresses. On the other hand, becoming rigid about any of these agreements will also create team problems. Just as in DBT treatment, perfection is not the goal; we are seeking a commitment and a stance that supports DBT and the team, an aspiration to meet these agreements. DBT providers are fallible! We expect team members will regularly struggle to meet these agreements; the team can nonjudgmentally seek solutions as needed, and even let some team problems go without intervention. As discussed multiple times throughout this book, flexibility is essential, and rigidity regarding these agreements will likely affect the team culture negatively.

DBT Assumptions about Clients and Therapy

Item 16 in the agreements refers to the DBT assumptions about clients and therapy, described in Chapter 1. As part of providing DBT, each DBT provider agrees to take a particular stance toward clients, each other, and the treatment. These assumptions affect the way one thinks about the client and the treatment, and are therefore an essential component of the DBT team. These are assumptions, not facts; they cannot be proven or debated in a factual way. Instead, it is a *choice* to believe these (as opposed to requiring proof) to improve one's effectiveness. An important component of the orientation and commitment discussion focuses on whether the potential team member is willing to embrace these assumptions. The clinical importance of these assumptions is discussed in Linehan (1993), and their relevance to team was discussed more fully in Chapter 1; here, they are listed as a reminder for the purposes of the orientation and commitment meeting.

DBT Assumptions about Clients

1. Clients are doing the best they can.
2. Clients want to improve.
3. Clients need to do better, try harder, and be more motivated to change.
4. Clients may not have caused all of their own problems, but they have to solve them anyway.
5. The lives of our clients can be unbearable.
6. Clients must learn new behaviors in all relevant contexts.
7. Clients cannot fail in therapy.
8. DBT team members need support.

DBT Assumptions about Therapy

1. The most caring thing a DBT provider can do is help clients change in ways that bring them closer to their own ultimate goals.
2. Clarity, precision, and compassion are of the utmost importance in the conduct of therapy.
3. The therapeutic relationship is a real relationship between equals.
4. Principles of behavior are universal, affecting DBT providers no less than clients.
5. DBT providers can fail.
6. The treatment can fail even when DBT providers do not.

Commitment Strategies

Once the potential team member is oriented to the team agreements, commitment strategies can be utilized. These strategies are the same that are used in DBT therapy. They can also be used with an existing member whose commitment to one or more of the team agreements is waning. These strategies are implemented to facilitate voluntary membership in the team. At the same time, it is important not to convince someone to join or to exaggerate the pros of joining the team just to get them to agree. The team will only benefit from inviting those who will throw themselves into the culture of the team wholeheartedly.

The DBT commitment strategies* are:

- Selling the commitment: evaluating the pros and cons.
- Playing the devil's advocate.
- Connecting present commitment to prior commitment.
- Foot in the door/door in the face.
- Highlighting the freedom to choose and the absence of alternatives.
- Shaping.

Because individuals typically approach the team wanting to join, we can assume that they are willing and interested (although there may be exceptions to this, as with someone in an agency where attendance at a DBT team is mandatory, or someone offers to join without sufficient orientation). Therefore, with new team members, extensive commitment strategies are typically not necessary. The most commonly used DBT commitment strategies used in bringing on a new member are:

SELLING THE COMMITMENT: EVALUATING THE PROS AND CONS

With DBT clients, this involves examining the reasons why one might commit to treatment, and what cons that decision might introduce. As Linehan (1993) emphasizes, this helps the individual reflect upon the reasons why making the commitment is useful, as well as to develop counterarguments for potential problems in the commitment. Selling the idea of joining the team will likely not be necessary for someone who is approaching a team, but this strategy can be very useful to highlight the challenges of being on a DBT team and ensure the new member has fully

---

*See Linehan (1993) for a full description.

considered the pros and cons before joining. Typically, this discussion strengthens a new team member's commitment to the team, but it may also highlight reluctance or hesitation. Pros and cons can also be used when an existing member's behavior drifts away from a specific agreement; for example, if a team member becomes more judgmental in the team over time, other team members may review the pros and cons of a nonjudgmental stance, in an effort to reestablish a commitment to that agreement.

PLAYING THE DEVIL'S ADVOCATE

Commitment may also be strengthened with the devil's advocate strategy. This strategy involves arguing against the new member's commitment to the team, which often functions to deepen the commitment to the team. This is not used as a paradoxical technique, however; it is used in a transparent, genuine manner, to explore the new member's understanding and motivation to join the team. For example, one member may say to an applicant to the team, "This is really challenging. You've agreed to join pretty quickly, but I want to be sure you understand that it can be hard. We share mistakes with each other, and we show emotion in team. And we really prioritize team time, we don't double-book our team time and we all work hard to be there every week. It may not be like other teams you've been on. Why would you want to join a team like that?" If this discussion leads to someone realizing it is not the right time, it will be helpful to the team to identify that before the individual actually joins the team. Alternatively, if the person acknowledges the challenges and still wants to join the team, the individual will enter the team with a deeper commitment and understanding.

CONNECTING PRESENT COMMITMENT TO PRIOR COMMITMENTS

This strategy is helpful when a team member has previously expressed commitment to DBT, such as their desire to help challenging clients. Tying commitment to the DBT team to these previously established commitments can help to strengthen dedication to the team. This strategy can also be used when an existing team member's commitment has weakened; team members can strengthen the commitment oftentimes by referring to previous commitments made to the team and/or clients.

For example, if a team member says that getting to team on time is too difficult, reminding them of previously expressed commitment to punctuality can again strengthen the willingness to be punctual again. (This also highlights the importance of gaining the original commitment, so the team can refer back to that commitment if it wanes in the future.)

DBT has several other commitment strategies; they are typically less useful in a team context but may be implemented at times when a team member's commitment to team fades over time. Foot in the door, door in the face, highlighting the freedom to choose and the absence of alternatives, and shaping may all become relevant at some point in a team member's tenure but are less commonly used when one is joining the team.

TROUBLESHOOTING

Troubleshooting is a necessary component of the commitment phase; it is the process of identifying and solving the ways in which the agreement and plan can go awry once commitment is obtained. Simply asking, "What might get in the way?" can help one be mindful of potential threats to the plan. This is extremely helpful in averting and solving future problems. This commitment discussion is an ideal opportunity to openly explore where the individual may run into frustration, anxiety, willfulness, or other obstacles regarding these commitments (e.g., predicting one will have difficulty experiencing corrective feedback or making oneself vulnerable with teammates). The new member can be better prepared for the obstacles joining the team may present, and will have considered solutions in advance.

Assigning Team Roles

The topic of roles in a DBT team was discussed extensively in Chapters 2 and 3. In brief, DBT teams typically benefit from a team leader; if the team has not done so already, the team can have a discussion about the necessity of a team leader before additional members are recruited and the team begins running regular team meetings. Teams will also decide how to structure the roles of meeting leader, observer, and any additional roles the team deems useful. The structure of these roles may evolve over time; teams will need to make a mindful decision about which roles are needed in the team's early meetings to establish the team's culture and norms.

Moving to Regular Team Meetings and Maintenance

Once the team has completed the eight steps outlined above, it is time to move on to regular team meetings. This transition may be clearly demarcated in some teams; in others, it may be a more gradual transition, moving from team development and training to the maintenance of therapy for the therapist, the culture of the team, and fidelity to DBT.

Conclusion

Just as in DBT therapy, the commitment phase and establishment of precedents in DBT team is invaluable in paving the way for success. These steps are designed to facilitate the development and maintenance of fidelity to the treatment. While each team is different and may need to shape these steps to meet their own needs, neglecting these steps can lead to more difficulty later in the team's evolution. Navigating these topics early should enable the team to better maintain the DBT culture.

IDEAS FOR PRACTICE

- Discuss each member's training needs and goals and how the team might facilitate meeting those goals.
- Choose a team agreement and discuss it with team members. Identify challenges in your team with respect to that agreement. Discuss if any additions to the agreements may be helpful for your team.
- Discuss inclusion and exclusion criteria for the clients your team will treat.
- Practice orienting a family member or non-DBT colleague to the DBT team.
- Discuss the assumptions for clients and therapy in team. Identify which assumptions are more difficult for you. Discuss how incorporating the assumptions has helped you work with a client more effectively.

- Practice commitment strategies with teammates regarding their commitment to team and for any other commitments that might present a chance to practice.
- Have each member trouble-shoot a potential obstacle to maintaining the team agreements. This exercise might include team size; the time, location, or length of the team meeting; and any other variables that may create challenges in running the DBT team.

Reproducible Handouts

HANDOUT 1. CORE DBT TEAM AGREEMENTS

1. **Dialectical Agreement.** The DBT team agrees to accept, at least pragmatically, a dialectical philosophy. There is no absolute truth; therefore, when polarities arise, the task is to search for the synthesis rather than for the truth. The dialectical agreement does not proscribe strong opinions, nor does it suggest that polarities are undesirable. Rather, it simply points to the direction team members agree to take when passionately held polar positions threaten to divide the team.

2. **Consultation-to-the-Client Agreement.** The DBT team agrees that team members do not serve as intermediaries for clients with other professionals, including other members of the team. The team agrees that clients will have more opportunity to learn when a DBT provider consults with clients on how to interact with other team members. When providers intervene on behalf of clients, clients lose that opportunity to learn to resolve problems themselves. Thus, when a clinician says things that are unhelpful or ineffective to the client, the task of the other team members is to help their clients cope with this provider's behavior, not necessarily to reform the provider. This does not mean that the team members do not conduct therapy for the therapist, plan treatment for their clients together, exchange information about the clients (including their problems with other members of the team), and discuss problems in treatment. DBT providers strive to provide such learning opportunities, and only intervene on behalf of clients when it is effective to do so.

3. **Consistency Agreement.** Failures in carrying out treatment plans can be problematic; at the same time, they present opportunities for clients to learn to deal with the real world. The job of the DBT team is not to provide a stress-free, perfect environment for clients. Thus, the DBT team, including all members of the team, agrees that consistency of team members with one another is not necessarily expected; each member does not have to teach the same thing, nor do all have to agree on what are "proper rules" for therapy. Team members can each make their own decisions about how to proceed in therapy, within the DBT frame. Similarly, although it can make for smooth sailing when all members of an institution, agency, or clinic communicate the rules accurately and

(continued)

Adapted from Linehan (1993, pp. 117–119). Copyright © The Guilford Press. Adapted by permission.

clearly, mix-ups are viewed as inevitable and isomorphic with the world we all live in. Any time a team member, team, or agency delivers treatment inconsistently (both in relation to other providers and to themselves), it is seen as a chance for clients (as well as team members) to practice the skills taught in DBT.

4. **Observing-Limits Agreement.** The team agrees that all members are to observe their own personal and professional limits. Furthermore, team members agree not to judge limits different from their own as too narrow or too broad, and instead determine if the limits are effective in a given situation. The team may suggest that a member broaden or narrow limits to become more effective, and at the same time will accept each other's differing limits without judgment. Team members will do their best to communicate their limits effectively to clients and teammates, and at the same time, clients are expected to ask about, learn, and accept providers' limits.

5. **Phenomenological Empathy Agreement.** DBT team members agree, all other things being equal, to search for nonpejorative or phenomenologically empathic interpretations of clients' behavior. The agreement is based on the fundamental assumption that clients are trying their best and want to improve, rather than to sabotage the therapy or "play games" with their provider. When a teammate is unable to come up with such an interpretation, other team members agree to assist in doing so, meanwhile also validating any frustration or other emotions that may arise for the provider. Thus, DBT team members agree to hold one another nonjudgmentally in the DBT frame. They agree to also search for a nonpejorative interpretation of the behavior of teammates, clients' family members, and any other relevant individuals, as well.

6. **Fallibility Agreement.** There is an explicit agreement in DBT team that all team members are fallible. Thus, there is little need to be defensive, since it is agreed ahead of time that team members have probably done whatever problematic things they are accused of. The task of the team is to apply DBT principles to one another, in order to help each member stay within DBT. As with clients, however, problem solving with team members must be balanced with validation of the inherent wisdom of their stances. Because, in principle, all team members are fallible, it is agreed that they will inevitably violate all of the agreements discussed here. When this is done, they will rely on one another to point out the polarity and will move on to search for the synthesis.

HANDOUT 2. EXPANDED LIST
OF DBT TEAM AGREEMENTS

1. Dialectical Agreement.

2. Consultation-to-the-Client Agreement.

3. Consistency Agreement.

4. Observing-Limits Agreement.

5. Phenomenological Empathy Agreement.

6. Fallibility Agreement.

7. Consider oneself part of a community of therapists treating a community of clients.

8. Provide "therapy for the therapist."

9. Provide DBT.

10. Conceptualize clients' and each other's behavior from a behavioral perspective.

11. Treat team meetings as importantly as any other therapy session.

12. Be available to fulfill the role for which one joined the team.

13. Be willing to call out the "elephant in the room" when others do not.

14. Remain one-mindful in team.

15. Assess sufficiently before offering solutions.

16. Strive to follow the assumptions about clients and therapy.

17. Follow team policy regarding providing coverage for each other, missing team, and missing appointments with clients.

18. Continue focusing on all of the above, even when feeling burned out, frustrated, tired, overworked, underappreciated, hopeless, ineffective, etc.

Adapted with permission from Marsha M. Linehan, unpublished, University of Washington Behavioral Research and Therapy Clinics.

HANDOUT 3. DBT ASSUMPTIONS ABOUT CLIENTS AND ABOUT THERAPY

DBT Assumptions about Clients

1. Clients are doing the best they can.
2. Clients want to improve.
3. Clients need to do better, try harder, and be more motivated to change.
4. Clients may not have caused all of their own problems, but they have to solve them anyway.
5. The lives of our clients can be unbearable.
6. Clients must learn new behaviors in all relevant contexts.
7. Clients cannot fail in therapy.
8. DBT team members need support.

DBT Assumptions about Therapy

1. The most caring thing a DBT provider can do is help clients change in ways that bring them closer to their own ultimate goals.
2. Clarity, precision, and compassion are of the utmost importance in the conduct of therapy.
3. The therapeutic relationship is a real relationship between equals.
4. Principles of behavior are universal, affecting DBT providers no less than clients.
5. DBT providers can fail.
6. The treatment can fail even when DBT providers do not.

"DBT Assumptions about Clients" adapted from Linehan (1993, pp. 117–119). Copyright © 1993 The Guilford Press. Adapted by permission. "DBT Assumptions about Therapy" adapted with permission from Marsha M. Linehan, unpublished, University of Washington Behavioral Research and Therapy Clinics.

HANDOUT 4. DBT TEAM OBSERVER REMINDERS

The observer rings the bell *lightly* when:

- A team member did not speak during team.
- Nonmindfulness; a team member did two things at once.
- A team member was late or unprepared.
- A team member was defensive.
- A team member made a judgmental or noncompassionate comment.
- Solutions were offered before sufficient problem definition/assessment occurred.
- A team member was treated as fragile; there was an elephant in the room that was not discussed.
- A dialectic went unresolved.

Adapted with permission from Marsha M. Linehan, unpublished, University of Washington Behavioral Research and Therapy Clinics.

HANDOUT 5. DBT TEAM
OBSERVER REMINDERS CHECKLIST

Date: _____ Observer name: _____

Check each of the boxes that apply.

❑ A team member did not speak during the team meeting.
❑ The behavior was highlighted.
❑ A brief chain analysis was conducted.
❑ Solutions were agreed upon.
❑ A commitment to implement a solution was elicited.

A team member was not one-mindful, doing two things at once (i.e., reading and listening; talking on the telephone; chatting out of turn with other team members).

❑ The observer rang the bell.
❑ This behavior was highlighted and blocked by the team.

A team member was late for the meeting.

❑ The behavior was highlighted.
❑ A chain analysis was conducted.
❑ Solutions were agreed upon.
❑ A commitment to implement a solution was elicited.

A team member was obviously unprepared.

❑ The behavior was highlighted.
❑ A chain analysis was conducted.
❑ Solutions were agreed upon.
❑ A commitment to implement a solution was elicited.

A team member displayed defensiveness in response to feedback.

❑ The observer rang the bell.
❑ The behavior was highlighted.
❑ The team member was asked to rephrase the statement(s).

(continued)

Adapted with permission from Marsha M. Linehan, unpublished, University of Washington Behavioral Research and Therapy Clinics.

A team member spoke in a judgmental or noncompassionate manner about his or her client(s), others, or themselves.

❑ The observer rang the bell.
❑ This behavior was highlighted and blocked by the team.
❑ The team member was asked to rephrase the judgmental statement(s).

A team member offered solutions before the problem was clearly defined.

❑ The observer rang the bell.
❑ The behavior was highlighted.
❑ The problem was clarified.

A team member was treated as "fragile." An obvious issue came up that needed to be targeted (e.g., defensiveness, judgmental talking, lateness) that was not highlighted or discussed by the team. Or, feedback clearly was needed, but was not provided.

❑ The observer rang the bell.
❑ The behavior was highlighted.
❑ The team discussed the avoided issue or provided the needed feedback.

A dialectic went unresolved.

❑ The observer rang the bell.
❑ The polarization was highlighted by the team.
❑ The other pole was sought out and explored.

HANDOUT 6. DBT TEAM NOTES: TEMPLATE 1

Notetaker: _____ Date: _____

Team members in attendance: _____

1. Team member of the week: _____
   a. Problem definition: _____
   b. Team feedback/ideas: _____

      _____

      _____

   c. Provider agreed to: _____

      _____

2. Team member: _____
   a. Problem definition: _____
   b. Team feedback/ideas: _____

      _____

      _____

   c. Provider agreed to: _____

      _____

3. Team member: _____
   a. Problem definition: _____
   b. Team feedback/ideas: _____

      _____

      _____

   c. Provider agreed to: _____

      _____

4. Team member: _____
   a. Problem definition: _____
   b. Team feedback/ideas: _____

      _____

      _____

   c. Provider agreed to: _____

      _____

Other items of note: _____

_____

_____

HANDOUT 7. DBT TEAM NOTES: TEMPLATE 2

Day of week:

Leader:

Observer:

Notetaker:

Attendees:

Absent:

FUNCTION OF TEAM (reminder): Monitoring and increasing team members' use of effective interventions, maintain and increase team members' motivation

Paperwork out of compliance (notes, intakes, termination reports):

Compliance plan:

ADMINISTRATIVE ISSUES:

EFFECTIVE BEHAVIOR (describe):

SKILLS GROUP UPDATE:

Leaders:

Present:

Absent:

Handout/page/topic reviewed:

Handout/page/topic taught:

Homework assigned:

Clinically significant notes:

OUT-OF-TOWN DATES:

CONSULTATION (repeat this section as needed):

Team member:

Problem/issue:

Comments/advice:

TEACHING POINTS:

TEAM FUNCTIONING (IDEAS/UPDATES):

Adapted with permission from Marsha M. Linehan, unpublished, University of Washington Behavioral Research and Therapy Clinics.

HANDOUT 8. DBT TEAM
CONFIDENTIALITY AGREEMENT

Confidentiality Agreement for Members of the DBT Team

Communications between DBT providers and their clients are considered to be confidential, and privileged from disclosure, as long as these communications are made in the course of diagnosis or treatment.

To have the most effective therapy possible, I understand and agree that I am seeking therapeutic treatment from other licensed providers during consult sessions. During these sessions, I am seeking treatment as a client of my colleagues, and when needed, offering my professional therapy services to other colleagues that are acting as clients to me. I understand and agree that as long as the consult meetings among DBT providers are held with providers acting in their professional roles of therapist to one another to further one's diagnosis or treatment, then the privilege also covers the consult team meetings.

I agree to maintain confidentiality of all words, conduct, and other communications, verbal and nonverbal, expressed during these consult meetings, including anything related to video/audio recordings. I recognize that effective psychotherapy depends upon an atmosphere of confidence and trust so that all group members feel comfortable to make frank and complete disclosures of facts, emotions, memories, and fears.

As a member of this group, **I agree not to disclose to anyone outside the group any confidential information that may help to identify another group member.** This includes, but is not limited to, names, physical descriptions, biological information, and specifics to the content of interactions with other group members. **I understand that I may be required to disclose confidential information for legal or ethical reasons, and team members may be required to disclose such information about me.**

By my signature below, I acknowledge that I have read carefully and understand the Team Agreement and that I agree to its terms and conditions.

Signature: _____

Name (Printed): _____

Date: _____

Adapted with permission from Marsha M. Linehan, unpublished, University of Washington Behavioral Research and Therapy Clinics.

HANDOUT 9. DBT TEAM
MEETING AGENDA: TEMPLATE 1

Team member indicates a need for one or more of the following when speaking to the team:

(1) Validation from the team

(2) Help increasing empathy toward client

(3) Help improving assessment with client

(4) Problem-solving suggestions

Check box when topic has been discussed/completed.

❑ Mindfulness

❑ Read agreement

❑ Review last week's notes

❑ Reminders to place on the agenda if more help is needed:
- Who is treating someone at high risk for imminent suicide?
- Who is treating a potential four-misses person?
- Who is going out of town?
- Who has out-of-date paperwork?
- Who is treating someone who is doing worse?
- Who has a client coming to the end of the treatment agreement?
- Who spent a lot of time on the phone this week?
- Was anyone late to team today?

❑ Group updates (which skill was taught, homework assigned, upcoming skill)

❑ Team member of the week: _____

15 minutes spent on one of the following: (1) role play, (2) viewing video, (3) presenting case formulation

PRIORITIZATION:

High priority (e.g., life-threatening behavior, high team member distress, time-sensitive topics, important team-interfering behaviors)
Team member initials:

❑ _____   ❑ _____

❑ _____   ❑ _____

Medium priority (e.g., topics that are important but not time sensitive, it's OK if we run out of time today)

❑ _____   ❑ _____

❑ _____   ❑ _____

Low priority (e.g., topics that can wait; there is a fair chance that these topics may get skipped today)

❑ _____   ❑ _____

❑ _____   ❑ _____

Other:

❑ Effective client or team member behaviors/progress _____

❑ Ring bell to end meeting

Adapted with permission from Marsha M. Linehan, unpublished, University of Washington Behavioral Research and Therapy Clinics.

HANDOUT 10. DBT TEAM
MEETING AGENDA: TEMPLATE 2

Date: _____ Leader: _____

Check box when topic has been discussed/completed.

❑ Mindfulness (10 minutes)

❑ Read agreement

❑ Review last week's notes

❑ Skills update on whiteboard

❑ REMINDERS: if you need help with the following, please put on the agenda:

✓ A client who is at a higher risk for suicide?
✓ A client who is at risk of missing four sessions in a row?
✓ A need for back-up coverage for travel?
✓ Paperwork requirements that are out of date?
✓ A client who is engaging in increasingly ineffective behaviors?
✓ A client near the end of the treatment period?
✓ Spent a lot of time phone coaching this week?
✓ Was anyone late to team today?

Place your initials on the agenda. (Remember to put the *team member* on the agenda.)

Check box for what you need today. Indicate priority and minutes needed.

Number of minutes requested	Priority: 1–5 (5 = highest)	Team member initials		I need help with ASSESSMENT	I need help with PROBLEM SOLVING	I need help building EMPATHY for my client	I need VALIDATION	I am BURNED OUT (please define for team)	I have an UPDATE	I DON'T KNOW what I need, but I need HELP!	I have an ANNOUNCEMENT

Adapted with permission from the Evidence Based Treatment Centers of Seattle.

References

Aarons, G. A., Sommerfeld, D. H., Hecht, D. B., Silovsky, J. F., & Chaffin, M. J. (2009). The impact of evidence-based practice implementation and fidelity monitoring on staff turnover: Evidence for a protective effect. *Journal of Consulting and Clinical Psychology, 77*(2), 270–280.

Addis, M., & Martell, C. (2004). *Overcoming depression one step at a time: The new behavioral activation approach to getting your life back.* Oakland, CA: New Harbinger.

Bateman, A. W., & Fonagy, P. (2004). Mentalization-based treatment of BPD. *Journal of Personality Disorders, 18*(1), 36–51.

Brent, D. A., Poling, K. D., & Goldstein, T. R. (2011). *Treating depressed and suicidal adolescents: A clinician's guide.* New York: Guilford Press.

Castelli Dransart, D. A., Heeb, J. L., Gulfi, A., & Gutjahr, E. (2015). Stress reactions after a patient suicide and their relations to the profile of mental health professionals. *BMC Psychiatry, 15*(265), 1–9.

Chugani, C. D., Mitchell, M. E., Botanov, Y., & Linehan, M. M. (2017). Development and initial evaluation of the psychometric properties of the Dialectical Behavior Therapy Barriers to Implementation Scale (BTI-S). *Journal of Clinical Psychology, 73,* 1704–1716.

Craske, M. G., Treanor, M., Conway, C. C., Zbozinek, T., & Vervliet, B. (2014). Maximizing exposure therapy: An inhibitory learning approach. *Behaviour Research and Therapy, 58,* 10–23.

DeRubeis, R. J., & Feeley, M. (1990). Determinants of change in cognitive therapy for depression. *Cognitive Therapy and Research, 14*(5), 469–482.

Draper, B., Kolves, K., DeLeo, D., & Snowdon, J. (2014). The impact of patient suicide and sudden death on health care professionals. *General Hospital Psychiatry, 36*(6), 721–725.

Gulfi, A., Castelli Dransart, D. A., Heeb, J. L., & Gutjahr, E. (2015). The impact of patient suicide on the professional reactions and practices of mental health caregivers and social workers. *Crisis, 31,* 202–210.

Haga, E., Aas, E., Groholt, B., Tormoen, A. J., & Mehlum, L. (2018). Cost-effectiveness of dialectical behaviour therapy vs. enhanced usual care in the treatment of adolescents with self harm. *Child and Adolescent Psychiatry and Mental Health, 12*(22), 1–11.

Hendin, H., Lipschitz, A., Maltsberger, J. T., Haas, A. P., & Wynecoop, S. (2000). Therapist's reactions to patients' suicides. *American Journal of Psychiatry, 157*(12), 2022–2027.

Katz, L., & Korslund, K. (in press). Principles of behavioral assessment and management of "life-threatening behavior" in dialectical behavior therapy. *Cognitive and Behavioral Practice.*

Koerner, K. (2012). *Doing dialectical behavior therapy: A practical guide.* New York: Guilford Press.

Koerner, K., & Linehan, M. M. (1997). Case formulation in dialectical behavior therapy for borderline personality disorder. In T. D. Elles (Ed.), *Handbook of psychotherapy case formulation* (pp. 340–367). New York: Guilford Press.

Krawitz, R., & Miga, E. M. (2019). Financial cost-effectiveness of dialectical behaviour therapy (DBT) for borderline personality disorder (BPD). In M. A. Swales (Ed.), *The Oxford handbook of dialectical behaviour therapy.* New York: Oxford University Press.

Kristensen, T. S., Borritz, M., Villadsen, E., & Christensen, K. B. (2005). The Copenhagen Burnout Inventory: A new tool for the assessment of burnout. *Work and Stress, 19,* 192–207.

Linehan, M. M. (1993). *Cognitive-behavioral treatment of borderline personality disorder.* New York: Guilford Press.

Linehan, M. M. (1997). Validation and psychotherapy. In A. Bohart & L. Greenberg (Eds.), *Empathy reconsidered: New directions in psychotherapy* (pp. 353–392). Washington, DC: American Psychological Association.

Linehan, M. M. (2015a). *DBT skills training handouts and worksheets* (2nd ed.). New York: Guilford Press.

Linehan, M. M. (2015b). *DBT skills training manual* (2nd ed.). New York: Guilford Press.

Linehan, M. M., Comtois, K. A., & Ward-Ciesielski, E. F. (2012). Assessing and managing risk with suicidal individuals. *Cognitive and Behavioral Practice, 19*(2), 218–232.

Linehan, M. M., & Heard, H. (1999). Borderline personality disorder: Costs, course, and treatment outcomes. In N. Miller & K. Magruder (Eds.), *The cost-effectiveness of psychotherapy: A guide for practitioners, researchers and policy-makers* (pp. 291–305). New York: Oxford University Press.

Maslach, C., & Jackson, S. E. (1981). The measurement of experienced burnout. *Journal of Occupational Behaviour, 2,* 99–113.

Novotney, A. (2016). 5 ways to avoid malpractice. *Monitor on Psychology, 47*(3), 5.

Pasieczny, N., & Connor, J. (2011). The effectiveness of dialectical behaviour therapy in routine public mental health settings: An Australian controlled trial. *Behaviour Research and Therapy, 49*(1), 4–10.

Ramnerö, J., & Törneke, N. (2008). *The ABCs of human behavior.* Oakland, CA: Context Press/New Harbinger.

Rizvi, S. L., & Sayrs, J. H. R. (in press). Assessment-driven case formulation and treatment planning in dialectical behavior therapy: Using principles to guide effective treatment. *Cognitive and Behavioral Practice.*

Rizvi, S. L., Steffel, L. M., & Carson-Wong, A. (2013). An overview of dialectical behavior therapy for professional psychologists. *Professional Psychology:
Research and Practice, 44*(2), 73–80.

Ruskin, R., Safinofsky, I., Bagby, R. M., Dickens, S., & Sousa, G. (2004). Impact of
patient suicide on psychiatrists and psychiatric trainees. *Academic Psychiatry,
28*(2), 104–110.

Saxe, G. N., Ellis, H. B., & Kaplow, B. (2007). *Collaborative treatment of traumatized
children and teens: The trauma systems therapy approach*. New York: Guilford
Press.

Sayrs, J. H. R. (2019). Running an effective DBT consultation team: Principles and
challenges. In M. A. Swales (Ed.), *The Oxford handbook of dialectical behavior
therapy*. New York: Oxford University Press.

Sayrs, J. H. R., & Linehan, M. M. (2019). Modifying CBT to meet the challenge of
treating emotion dysregulation: Utilizing dialectics. In M. A. Swales (Ed.), *The
Oxford handbook of dialectical behavior therapy*. New York: Oxford University
Press.

Sitkin, S. B., & Lind, E. A. (2007). *The six domains of leadership: A new model for
developing and assessing leadership qualities*. Chapel Hill, NC: Delta Leadership.

Sitkin, S. B., Lind, E. A., & Siang, S. (2006, Fall). The six domains of leadership.
Leader to Leader, 2006(S1), 27–33.

Sung, J. (2016a). Sample agency practices for responding to client suicide. Retrieved
from *www.sprc.org/sites/default/files/resource-program/Sample_Agency_Practices.
pdf*.

Sung, J. (2016b). Sample individual practitioner practices for responding to client
suicide. Retrieved from *www.sprc.org/sites/default/files/resource-program/Sample_
Individual_Practitioner_Practices.pdf*.

Swales, M. A., & Dunkley, C. (2019). Structuring the wider environment and the
DBT team: Skills for DBT team leads. In M. A. Swales (Ed.), *The Oxford handbook of dialectical behaviour therapy*. New York: Oxford University Press.

U.S. Department of Health and Human Services. (2013). Health information of
deceased individuals. Retrieved from *www.hhs.gov/hipaa/for-professionals/
privacy/guidance/health-information-of-deceased-individuals/index.html*.

Index

Note. *f* following a page number indicates a figure.